REMARKS ON THE USES

OF SOME OF THE

BAZAAR MEDICINES

AND

COMMON MEDICAL PLANTS OF INDIA

REMARKS ON THE USES

OF SOME OF THE

BAZAAR MEDICINES

AND

COMMON MEDICAL PLANTS OF INDIA

WITH A FULL INDEX OF DISEASES, INDICATING THEIR
TREATMENT BY THESE AND OTHER AGENTS
PROCURABLE THROUGHOUT INDIA.

EDWARD JOHN WARING, C. I. E., M.D.

GYAN

Published by

Gyan Publishing House
5, Ansari Road
Daryaganj, New Delhi-110002
Phone: 011-47034999, 9811692060
E-mail: books@gyanbooks.com

Distribution Network
gyanbooks.com
India, USA, Canada, UK, Australia, France

ISBN : 978-81-212-9544-4 (PB)
First Published, 1883

2nd Impression 2023

Printed at: Gyan Press, Delhi.

REMARKS ON THE USES OF SOME OF THE BAZAAR MEDICINES AND COMMON MEDICAL PLANTS OF INDIA

Author: EDWARD JOHN WARING

REMARKS ON THE USES

OF SOME OF THE

BAZAAR MEDICINES

AND

COMMON MEDICAL PLANTS OF INDIA.

REMARKS ON THE USES

OF SOME OF THE

BAZAAR MEDICINES

AND

COMMON MEDICAL PLANTS OF INDIA

WITH A FULL INDEX OF DISEASES, INDICATING THEIR TREATMENT BY THESE AND OTHER AGENTS PROCURABLE THROUGHOUT INDIA.

TO WHICH ARE ADDED

DIRECTIONS FOR TREATMENT IN CASES OF DROWNING, SNAKE-BITES, &c.

BY

EDWARD JOHN WARING, C. I. E., M.D.

FELLOW OF THE ROYAL COLLEGE OF PHYSICIANS OF LONDON,
SURGEON-MAJOR (RETIRED) HER MAJESTY'S INDIAN ARMY,
EDITOR OF THE PHARMACOPŒIA OF INDIA, ETC.

Fourth Edition.

1883.

PREFACE

TO THE FOURTH EDITION.

THAT this little work should have reached a FOURTH EDITION may be taken as pretty clear indication that it has met a recognised want amongst our Indian fellow-subjects, for whose instruction and guidance it was originally issued. To render it worthy of continued favour, and to make it additionally useful, has been my anxious endeavour.

Of any merit which this edition may be found to possess over the preceding one, a very large portion is due to Dr. J. E. T. Aitchison, C. I. E., Surgeon-Major in H. M. Indian (Bengal) Medical Service, who, with a liberality that demands my warmest thanks, placed at my disposal an elaborate MS. commentary on the Third Edition, embodying his own professional experience in India (extending over many years), and supplying the vernacular names of the various drugs in the Punjábí, Kashmírí, and Leh languages. Of this document it need hardly be said I have availed myself largely, my only regret being that I could not insert it *in extenso*, but to have done this would greatly have exceeded the prescribed limits of the work. As it is, Dr. Aitchison has laid me under a vast obligation, which I am only too happy to have this opportunity of acknowledging.

Five new articles have been added to the List of Drugs: two at the suggestion of Dr. Aitchison; namely, (1) Sugar, and (2) Kerosine Oil, which latter, owing to its extensive use for lighting purposes during the past few years, is now obtainable in nearly every bazaar in the country; the other three being the (3) Cinchona Febrifuge (Quinetum), (4) Petroleum, and (5) Rock Salt. The various ways in which these articles may be utilised in the treatment of disease will be found under their respective headings in the 'Addenda,' p. 167, *et seq.*

In addition to these there have been introduced notices of Indian Hemp (Gunjah) smoking in the treatment of Tetanus, of the antiscorbutic properties of Ámchur (dried Mangoes), the lactifuge powers of Sambac flowers (*Jasminum Sambac*), the emmenagogue virtues of Til or Jinjili Seeds (*Sesamum Indicum*), and other points unnoticed in previous editions. The therapeutic applications of Water are enlarged upon; as also are those of Carbolic Acid, especially in the treatment of Leprosy. The Sick Dietary has likewise been extended. Amongst the new matter has been introduced a section (pp. 255–58) detailing the 'Precautions to be taken by persons residing in Snake-infested localities.'

By these and other additions (occupying upwards of thirty pages of new matter), and by the revision and modification of other passages, it is confidently hoped that the practical value of the work will be found to be materially increased. Indeed, it has been my earnest endeavour throughout to render this little volume as useful as possible, and if through its instrumentality suffering humanity be in any degree benefited my highest aspiration will be attained.

E. J. WARING.

PREFACE

TO THE SECOND EDITION.

FOURTEEN years have elapsed since this work, in an elementary form, was first issued for the use of the District Vaccinators of Travancore, whose sphere of action was far removed from regular medical aid. It was originally published in English and Tamil on opposite pages; subsequently it was reprinted in Tamil alone by the London Missionary Society's Press at Nagercoil, for the use of the catechists and others connected with that Mission. In 1868, a Malyalim translation, by Dresser Ramswammy Rajoo, was issued by the Travancore Government. From reports received from various quarters, there is reason to believe that the work has enjoyed a wide circulation amongst the people of Travancore and Tinnevelly, and that it has exercised a considerable influence on the practice of the native doctors of those districts.

Were I wise, I ought, perhaps, to rest satisfied with these results, which far exceed what were originally contemplated; but recent observation has convinced me that there are other classes scattered through our great Indian possessions, to whom a work of the kind would prove most acceptable, by pointing out to them the agents—either purchasable in the bazaars at an almost nominal price, or procurable at the cost of collection, from the road-sides, waste places, or gardens in the immediate neighbourhood of almost every out-station—by means of which, with the exercise of ordinary intelligence, they may often be enabled to relieve the sufferings of those amongst whom their lot has been cast.

And at the head of these classes stand the Missionaries, whose stations, for the most part, are too far removed from the busy haunts of men to allow of their calling in regular medical aid in cases of sickness, and who are consequently thrown, at such times, very much on their own resources. Many of the missionaries have under their charge large establishments of catechists, pupils, &c.; and it cannot be otherwise than highly desirable that they should be put in possession of any information regarding the available means of relieving the sufferings, and treating the diseases, of those placed under their care. This is not the place to enter into a disquisition on missionary work, but I cannot refrain from expressing my firm conviction that the more the principle of Medical Missions—making Religion and Medicine go hand in hand—is carried out, the greater, humanly speaking, will be the success of missionary efforts. How many a door for the admission of Gospel truth, which would otherwise be shut, would be opened, and that readily, to one who, with 'the glad tidings of great joy' in the one hand, would bring in the other the means of relieving physical suffering and curing bodily disease! The highest distinction that I would claim for this little work is, that it may constitute, as far as India is concerned, a Missionaries' Medical Vade Mecum.

Next on the *rôle* comes a large army of European and Anglo-Indian officials, whether within the magic circle of 'the Service' or beyond its pale, who are attached to the Public Works, Forests, Railway, Telegraph, or other Departments, or employed in Tea, Coffee, or Cotton plantations, in commercial pursuits, &c., many of them married men, with families and a large number of dependants, the majority at distant 'up-country stations,' miles away from medical aid; how important for persons under such circumstances to possess a knowledge of the means lying (literally so in many instances) at their very feet, by which pain and suffering may be alleviated, and, perhaps, a valuable life saved.

Lastly, but by no means least, either in point of numbers or importance, comes the daily increasing array of educated Natives, who, as a class, readily avail themselves of every scrap of knowledge drawn from trustworthy European sources, which tends to throw light on the products and resources of their native land. Whilst, on the one hand, I am perfectly prepared to admit that much of the knowledge I possess of the properties and uses of Indian drugs has been derived from Native sources, I think I may, on the other hand, without presumption, claim the credit of repaying the debt with interest, furnishing in return a considerable amount of information on the uses of even the same drugs, of which the Natives themselves had previously no idea. It is to this class that I venture to think this little work will prove most useful and acceptable.

In addition to the above, I venture to hope that to even duly qualified Medical Officers, especially at up-country stations, a work like the present may prove serviceable on emergencies, *e. g.*, a failure of the supply of European drugs, &c., by showing them what resources they have at command in the bazaars or in their immediate neighbourhood, by means of which many a gap may be stopped till more efficient remedies are available.

In undertaking a Second Edition of this work, I have been further influenced by a desire to render its scope and contents more complete. With more extended knowledge on my part, drawn partly from subsequent personal experience in the use of Indian drugs, and partly from the Reports received from Medical Officers during the preparation of the Pharmacopœia of India, I realised how imperfect the original work was; and feeling myself in a position to add much information which would tend to increase its usefulness, I determined upon issuing another edition. The whole work has accordingly been rewritten and greatly enlarged.

It was evidently quite out of the question, in a small work like the present, to include the host of medicines included under the general headings of 'Bazaar Medicines' and 'Common Medical Plants of India,' but from them I have made a selection of about 80, comprising—1 Antacid, 8 Astringents, 3 Antispasmodics, 2 Antiscorbutics, 6 Antiperiodics, 5 Demulcents and Emollients, 4 Diaphoretics or Sudorifics, 4 Diuretics, 3 Expectorants, 2 Emmenagogues, 4 Emetics, 6 Purgatives, 3 Narcotics or Sedatives, 5 Refrigerants, 9 Stomachics or Carminatives, 7 Bitter Tonics, 5 Alterative Tonics or Alteratives, 2 Metallic Tonics, 7 Local and 4 General Stimulants, 2 Vesicants, or Blistering Agents, 6 Vermifuges, and 17 Miscellaneous Articles, not included in the above classes.

In making this selection I have been guided by the following principles:—1. By the safety of the drug; hence Arsenic, Aconite Root (Bish), Nux Vomica, Indian Hemp,. and some other powerful medicines have been omitted, as it was felt to be inadvisable, in a work like the present, to introduce agents which, in the hands of unprofessional persons, might do more harm than good if employed in unsuitable cases. Where, however, a powerful drug, *e. g.* Opium, has been admitted, minute directions as to its employment have been given. 2. By the acknowledged utility or efficacy of the drug as proved by European experience. 3. By the drug possessing a generally well-known, recognised native name. 4. By its wide distribution and easy procurability in all parts, and in all the bazaars of India generally. It is hoped that by the addition of the native names and descriptions of the drugs (which were omitted in the First Edition), even a new-comer will have little difficulty in obtaining and recognising any particular article he may require.

With this native 'Apparatus Medicaminum' very much may be accomplished under ordinary circumstances, in the way of relieving suffering and curing disease; but it must be admitted that there are certain articles included under the class 'European Medicines' for which the Indian bazaars supply no adequate substitutes. I have therefore (in Appendix C) added a list of nine drugs which it appears desirable should always be kept in store. They are— 1. Sulphate of Quinine; 2. Ipecacuanha; 3. Smyrna, or Turkey Opium; 4. Calomel; 5. Acetate of Lead;

6. Santonin; 7. Liquor Ammoniæ; 8. Blistering Fluid; and 9. Carbolic Acid.* No attempt has been made in the body of the work to enter into a description of the properties and uses of these drugs generally (with the exception of Opium), but in the Synopsis or Index of Diseases (Part II.) it has been pointed out how these valuable agents may be utilised in the most efficient manner. It is believed that, by adopting this course, the practical utility of the work will be greatly enhanced.

Attention is particularly directed to the Synopsis or Index of Diseases in Part II.; it is not pretended that the modes of treatment therein detailed are the best which could be adopted; the object has rather been to show how much good may be effected by the simple means at command at almost every 'up-country station' throughout India; and those who follow the directions may feel assured, that with the exercise of ordinary prudence, if they fail to do good they will at any rate do no harm.

It is advisable, however, in the treatment of the poorer and less enlightened class of Natives, such as constitute the mass of dispensary patients, to maintain a discreet silence as to the source from which the medicines are derived, as experience has shown that the Native poor soon cease to believe in European

* To these Bromide of Potassium and Biniodide of Mercury have since been added.

practice when they discover that they are being treated with Indian drugs. It is well, therefore, to disguise them with a little colouring matter, &c.

Notwithstanding the large amount of new matter incorporated in this edition, I am fully conscious of its numerous defects and shortcomings; hence I shall feel under an obligation to any of my medical and other friends in India who will favour me with any suggestions and observations (especially with reference to the use of Native drugs, drawn from personal experience), which would add to the practical value of future editions, should such be called for. All communications addressed to me, to the care of Messrs. GRINDLAY and Co., 55 Parliament Street, S.W., London, will be thankfully received.

LONDON, 1874.

INTRODUCTION.

THIS work, it is presumed, will fall into the hands of many who are wholly ignorant of, or very partially acquainted with, matters pharmaceutical; hence some few introductory remarks are indispensable to enable such persons to understand fully, and follow out correctly, the directions given.

1. *Weights and Measures.*—In Appendix C, a small set of Apothecaries' scales and weights is included, but in the absence of the former it is well to remember that a small set of scales, such as is used by native jewellers, can be procured for a few annas in every bazaar; care, however, is necessary to see that the balance is strictly correct and even.

Weights.—The Apothecary weights supplied from England have the following marks or signs impressed upon them:—

℈ſs	=	half a scruple	=	10 grains.
℈j	=	one scruple	=	20 „
ʒſs	=	half a drachm	=	30 „
ʒj	=	one drachm	=	60 „
ʒjſs	=	one drachm and a half	=	90 „
ʒij	=	two drachms	=	120 „

The small circular indentations on the grain weights indicate the number of grains each weight represents.

In the absence of these, the following hints may be useful :—

A new rupee of the present currency weighs 180 grains or three drachms.

A half rupee of the present currency weighs 90 grains or a drachm and a half.

A quarter rupee of the present currency weighs 45 grains or three quarters of a drachm.

To obtain smaller weights beat a new quarter rupee into a long, thin, narrow plate, and divide it carefully into three equal parts. You have thus three 15 grain weights. One of these divided again into three equal parts, furnishes three 5 grain weights. One of these subdivided into five equal parts furnishes five 1 grain weights. Care should be taken to see that the parts are of equal weights, and each part should be marked with a figure to denote its weight. A native jeweller, at a very small cost, will readily carry out the above subdivision.

With these, you may obtain any small weights you require; thus, if you require nine grains, you use a 5 grain weight and four single grain weights. If you want a drachm weight (60 grains), you use a quarter rupee (45 grains) and a 15 grain weight, which makes exactly the 60 grains or one drachm. To get a scruple (20 grains) weight, you use one of the 15 grain and one of the 5 grain weights = 20 grains or one scruple.

Two rupees and a half rupee together weigh 450 grains or slightly over one ounce, which weight they may be taken to represent, in the absence of regular weights in making up any of the prescriptions given in the following pages.

Measures of Capacity.—For these, the English Graduated Measures, glasses included, in Appendix C, should be employed. The marks on them signify as follows :—

♏	=	1 minim.
f℈j one fluid-drachm	=	60 minims.
f℥j one fluid-ounce	=	8 fluid-drachms.
O one pint	=	20 fluid-ounces.

In default of a graduated measure glass, it may be useful to know that a small cup of silver or other metal, exactly the circumference of a quarter rupee and 3¾ inches deep, will hold exactly one ounce, and twenty of these full of liquid make one pint. Each ounce contains eight fluid-drachms, so with the aid of this ounce measure you can calculate the quantity required pretty accurately. The measure should be made of silver, as some medicines, especially the acids, act on the other metals.

Any native jeweller would manufacture one of these measures in a short time, and at a very small cost.

In the following pages other domestic measures, as they may be termed, are mentioned; they represent approximately the following quantities :—

A wine-glassful (ordinary size) = one fluid-oz. & a half.

Two table-spoonfuls	...	= one oz.
One table-spoonful	...	= half oz.
One dessert-spoonful	...	= two drachms.
One tea-spoonful	...	= one drachm.

'A drop' may be taken generally to represent a minim, though in many instances they differ considerably in capacity.

It must be borne in mind that these measurements apply solely to fluids — never to solids. A table-spoonful of some solids, as powders, would *weigh* two or three ounces, whilst of others it might only be as many drachms.

Preparations.—A few hints on these may be useful to the uninitiated. *Infusions.*—In preparing these, the following points require attention: *a*, the solid ingredients should be cut into small pieces or slices, or bruised in a mortar, so that the water shall readily penetrate into the substance; *b*, the water should be *boiling; c*, the vessel or chattie containing the ingredients on which the boiling water has been poured, should be covered over to prevent evaporation, and set aside till the liquid is cold, when it should be strained through a muslin or thin rag. In hot climates infusions soon spoil, hence they should be freshly prepared every other day at the furthest. *Decoctions.*— These differ from Infusions so far that the ingredients are subject to the process of boiling. The requisite quantity of water having been heated to boiling-point, the solid ingredients, prepared as for infusions, are to be introduced, and the whole boiled in a covered vessel for the specified period. The liquid whilst hot should be strained and set aside in a covered vessel till cold. Like infusions, they rapidly become spoiled in hot climates. *Tinctures.*— These are formed by macerating the solid ingredients, prepared as directed for Infusions, in a bottle with the specified quantity of spirit, for seven days or more, occasionally shaking the same to ensure the spirit acting thoroughly on the ingredients. At the end of the specified period it should be strained, and the clear liquid set aside in a cool place in well-stoppered bottles, for use. Great care is necessary to prevent evaporation; hence if a glass-stoppered bottle is used, softened wax should be carefully placed round the stopper, which should be further secured by a cap of thin leather or wax-cloth tied tightly over it. It is thought by many that evaporation of spirit takes place less rapidly in a closely fitting *corked* bottle than in one provided with a glass stopper.* In either case layers of wax and the leather are advisable. Under the most favourable circumstances evaporation to a greater or lesser extent will take place in hot climates; hence by long keeping, the tincture acquires increased strength, and in regulating the dose of the more active tinctures, as of Opium or Datura, the fact ought to be borne in mind, or serious consequences may ensue. *Powders.*—When an article is ordered to be taken in the form of powder, it should be pulverised as finely

* Very serviceable corks, especially for temporary use, may be made out of Sola, the material used for hats, &c.

as possible. There is little difficulty in this when a large quantity of the article is required to be kept in store, as is generally advisable, as the natives, by the aid of the simple machinery which they employ in making 'Curry powder,' will reduce the hardest woody ingredients to the requisite state of fineness. When only a few grains or a small quantity is required, it may be obtained by means of a nutmeg-grater (included in List in Appendix C.), and subsequently triturating the rough powder thus obtained in a mortar till it is reduced to the state of a fine powder. In the preparation of a *Compound Powder*, *i. e.*, a powder containing two or more ingredients, it is of the greatest importance that they should be uniformly and thoroughly incorporated, else it is evident that a small portion of it, such as is usually prescribed as a dose, may contain an excess of one ingredient—it may be an active or dangerous one, and operate powerfully—whilst the next dose may be comparatively inert. Powders, when prepared in large quantities, should be kept in well-stoppered or corked bottles; if left in open vessels exposed to the action of the air, they soon become deteriorated. *Pills.*—For the reasons just stated, it is necessary, when two or more ingredients enter into the composition of a pill mass, to be careful that they are thoroughly incorporated. When powders, &c., enter into their composition, a little honey or jaggery is the best thing to give them cohesion and consistence. They should be moderately hard; if too soft, they are apt to lose the globular form which they ought to possess, and become a shapeless mass. When several pills are made, a little Arrowroot or Rice Flour should be added to the box which contains them, to keep them from adhering to one another. No pill should ordinarily exceed 5 grains in weight, otherwise there will be a difficulty in swallowing it; two 3 grain pills are more easily taken than one of 6 grains. Pills, when prepared in any quantity, should, like powders, be kept in well-stoppered or corked bottles.

Ointments.—Animal fats, *e. g.*, Lard which is so generally used in English pharmacy, are apt to become rancid and irritating in hot climates; hence they should be discarded in tropical practice. In India there is another cogent reason for abandoning them, viz., the religious prejudices of the natives, especially of the Mussulman, to whom hog's fat is an abomination. The only allowable animal fat in India is freshly prepared Ghee, or clarified butter; but this in the hotter part of India is of too thin consistence for ordinary ointments. Fortunately India supplies at least two vegetable substitutes, Kokum Butter and Piney Tallow (the expressed Oil of Vateria Indica). In addition to these, I have introduced a third article, Ceromel (a mixture of wax and honey). With these three agents it is believed that animal fats may be altogether dispensed with in Indian pharmacy.

Native Names.—These have been mainly derived from Mr. Moodeen Sheriff's valuable Catalogue, which forms the Supplement to the Pharmacopœia of India. Some have been drawn from Ainslie's *Materia Indica*, a work of sterling merit. For the Malay names I am indebted to the Hon. Major F. M'Nair, C.M.G., Surveyor-

General, Straits Settlements, and for the Punjábí and Kashmirí names to Dr. J. E. T. Aitchison, formerly British Commissioner, Ladakh.

It is only necessary, in this place, to indicate the pronunciation of the vowels met with in this work.

a (short) as in *a*bout, or the final *a* in Calcutt*a*.
á (long) as in *a*ll, c*a*ll.
e (short) as in *e*lbow, or the first *e* in n*e*ver.
é (long) as *a* in *a*ble or *ai* in f*ai*r.
i (short) as *i* in *i*nk, b*i*d.
í (long) as *ee* in f*ee*d and fr*ee*.
o (short) as in fr*o*m.
ó (long) as in *o*pium, h*o*me.
u (short) as in f*u*ll, or as in wolf.
ú (long) as in f*oo*l, t*oo*.

Explanation of the Abbreviations employed in the lists of the native names of the drugs :—

Hind. Hindústaní.
Duk. Dukhní.
Beng. Bengálí.
Punj. Punjábí.
Kash. Kashmirí.
Tam. Tamil.
Tel. Telugu.
Mal. Malyalim.
Can. Canarese.
Mah. Máhrattí.
Guz. Guzrattí.
Cing. Cingalese.
Burm. Burmese.
Malay. Malay.

REMARKS ON THE USES

OF SOME OF THE

BAZAAR MEDICINES OF INDIA.

PART I.

ALPHABETICAL LIST OF THE BAZAAR MEDICINES AND INDIAN MEDICAL PLANTS INCLUDED IN THIS WORK.

1. **Abelmoschus, or Edible Hibiscus. Okra.** The fresh unripe capsules or fruit of Abelmoschus (Hibiscus) esculentus, *Linn.*

Bhindí, Rám-turáí (*Hind.*), Bhéndí (*Duk.*, *Punj.*), Dhéras or Dhénras, Rám-toráí (*Beng.*), Vendaik-káy (*Tam.*), Benda-káya (*Tel.*), Ventak-káya (*Mal.*), Bendé-káyi (*Can.*), Bhéndá (*Mah.*), Bhíndu (*Guz.*), Banda-ká (*Cing.*), Youn-padi-sí (*Burm.*), Kachang-lindir (*Malay*).

2. This well-known vegetable, cultivated throughout India, abounds in a copious, bland, viscid mucilage, which possesses valuable emollient and demulcent properties, rendering the practitioner in India independent of mallow and other European articles of that class. The dried fruit may be employed where it

is not procurable in a fresh state. It is best given in decoction, prepared by boiling three ounces of the fresh capsules, cut transversely, in a pint and a half of water for twenty minutes, straining and sweetening to taste. This, taken as an ordinary drink, proves alike agreeable and serviceable in *Fevers, Catarrhal attacks, Irritable states of the Bladder and Kidneys,* in *Gonorrhœa,* and in *all cases attended with scalding pain, and difficulty in passing Urine.* Under its use the urine is said to become much increased in quantity. *In Dysentery,* especially in the chronic form of the disease, the bland viscid mucilage is often most beneficial. It is a good plan to give it in soup.

3. *In Hoarseness, and in dry and irritable states of the Throat, giving rise, as is often the case, to a troublesome Cough, as in Consumption, &c.,* the free inhalation of the vapour of the hot decoction (*ante*) has in many instances been found serviceable.

4. The fresh capsules bruised are stated to form an efficient emollient poultice.

5. **Abrus, or Country Liquorice Root.** The root of Abrus precatorius, *Linn.*

Mulatthí-hindi, Gunj-ka-jar (*Hind., Duk.*), Jaishtomodhu-bengala, Kunch-ka-jar (*Beng.*), Aslassús, Múlathí (*Punj.*), Shangir (*Kash.*), Gundumani-vér (*Tam.*), Guru-venda-véru (*Tel.*), Kunnikuru-véra (*Mal.*), Gul-ganji-béru (*Can.*), Olindamúl (*Cing.*), Yu-e-si-anú (*Burm.*), Akar-sagamerah (*Malay*).

6. This root, obtained from a twining shrub common throughout India, whose bright scarlet seeds with a black spot at one end are universally known, possesses many of the sensible properties and medical qualities of the true liquorice-root (which is also to be met with in some of the large bazaars), hence its common name, Country Liquorice. Properly prepared, and according to directions in Indian Pharmacopœia, it yields an extract similar to officinal liquorice, but less sweet and more bitter.* The following syrup has been found useful in the *Coughs of Childhood.* Take of fresh Abrus roots, the larger sized the better, well bruised, two ounces; and Abelmoschus capsules sliced, one ounce; boil in a pint of water for half an hour, and strain; to the liquor add eight ounces of sugar-candy or honey, and boil down to the consistence of a syrup. From a tea to a table-spoonful may be freely given several times a day when the cough is troublesome, whether fever is present or not. It forms also a good adjunct to other more active cough mixtures. The great objection to this, in common with all syrups in India, is the readiness with which it undergoes

* According to Moodeen Sheriff (*Suppl. to Ind. Ph.*, p. 18), an extract prepared from the dried leaves of Abrus precatorius is much superior both in taste and as a medicine to that prepared from the root. He gives the following directions for its preparation:—Pour boiling distilled water on the dried leaves till they are sufficiently covered; keep the vessel on a slow fire for six hours; then strain the liquor while hot through flannel and evaporate on a water bath to a proper consistence. The extract prepared from the juice of the fresh leaves, he adds, is also sweet, but very inferior to the latter for medicinal purposes.

fermentation; hence only small quantities should be prepared when cases occur requiring its use.

7. **Acacia, or Babúl Bark.** The bark of Acacia Arabica, *Willd.*

Babúl-ka-chál, Kíkar-ka-chál (*Hind.*), Kali-kíkar-kí chilká (*Duk.*), Babúl-sál (*Beng.*), Sák (*Punj.*, *Kash.*), Karu-vélam-pattai (*Tam.*), Kulit-pokoh-bunga (*Malay*).

8. Babúl bark occurs in large thick pieces, coarsely fibrous, of a deep mahogany colour, and astringent, bitterish taste. It is an excellent astringent, and though less powerful than some others of the same class, it possesses the advantage of being obtainable, either in the fresh or dried state, throughout India, the tree yielding it being common everywhere in dry, sandy localities.

9. The best form for medical purposes is a decoction prepared by boiling one ounce and a half of the bruised bark in a pint of water for ten minutes, and straining. Of this the dose is from one and a half to two ounces twice daily, or oftener in *Chronic Diarrhœa*, &c.; it is, however, chiefly employed as an external or local application—as an injection in *Leucorrhœa and other Vaginal Discharges;* as an enema in *Piles* and *Prolapsus* (*Descent*) *of the Anus*, and as a gargle in *Sore Throat, and in Sponginess and Ulceration of the Gums.* In all these cases, however, it is generally used conjoined with alum and other agents.

10. **Acorus, or Sweet Flag Root.** The root stock or Acorus Calamus, *Linn.*

Bach or Vach (*Hind.*, *Duk.*), Bach, Saféd Bach (*Beng.*), Warch (*Punj.*) Vá'í (*Kash.*), Vashambú (*Tam.*), Vasa, Vadaja (*Tel.*), Vash-anpa (*Mal.*), Bajé (*Can.*), Vékhanda (*Mah.*), Vaj, Vach (*Guz.*), Lene or Linhe (*Burm.*), Jaringowe (*Malay*).

11. This is one of the commonest of bazaar medicines, and generally procurable everywhere, of good quality, at a very small cost. It occurs in pieces of various lengths, about the thickness of the thumb, rather flattened, spongy, provided with numerous sheath-like, ringed appendages; odour peculiar and aromatic; taste, bitterish, warm and somewhat acrid. Till very recently, it was included in the British Pharmacopœia. It well deserves a place in every Indian domestic medicine chest.

12. It is a tonic and stomachic of no small value, and is best given in the form of infusion : one ounce of the bruised root to half a pint of boiling water, in doses of a wine-glassful twice or thrice daily. Combined with Chiretta, it has been reported to cure *Intermittent Fevers in natives*, but though its power in this respect is doubtful, except, perhaps, in cases of the mildest description, yet in *Convalescence after this and other forms of Fever*, a mixture of equal parts of the infusion of Acorus and Chiretta (98) is as good a formula as can be employed. The same combination proves also most serviceable in *Dyspepsia, especially*

when attended with much flatulence, in Loss of Appetite and Constitutional Debility.

13. *In the Dysentery of Natives, and in that especially of Native Children,* Dr. Evers (*Indian Medical Gazette,* Feb. 1, 1875) speaks very highly of Acorus given in decoction as follows: Take of the bruised root-stock two ounces, Coriander seed one drachm, Black Pepper half a drachm, Water one pint; boil down to about twelve ounces (or for about a quarter of an hour), and set aside to cool. The dose for an adult is a wine-glassful three times daily; for a child from one to three tea-spoonfuls, sweetened with sugar, two or three times a-day. Astringents or Quinine (the latter when the disease is apparently of malarious origin) may be added if necessary. Dr. Evers found this decoction not only useful in *Dysentery and Diarrhœa,* but also in the *Bronchitic Affections of Children.* He considers it worthy of a more extended trial.

14. This root, especially when freshly collected, and retaining its full aroma, is reported, on good authority, to *drive away fleas and other insects,* a fact well to bear in mind in a sick room, as well as elsewhere.

15. **Aloes.** The inspissated juice of Aloe Socotrina, *Linn.*, and other species of Aloe.

Musabbar, Ilvá, Yalvá (*Hind.*), Musanbar (*Duk.*), Móshabbar (*Beng.*), Elwá (*Punj.*), Mússbar, Sibar (*Kash.*), Kariya-pólam, Irakta-pólam (*Tam.*), Múshámbaram (*Tel.*), Chenna-náyakam (*Mal.*),

Musam-bara-bóla (*Mah.*), Yéliyo (*Guz.*), Kalu-bólam, Kari-bolam (*Cing.*), Mo (*Burm.*), Jadam (*Malay*).

16. Aloes, as met with in the bazaars, is generally imported, and of a very inferior description, but it may be rendered fit for medical use by the following process: Take of bazaar Aloes, in small fragments, one pound; boiling water, one gallon; stir them well together until they are thoroughly mixed, and set aside for twelve hours; then pour off the clear liquor, strain the remainder, mix the liquors, and place in open vessels in the sun, or over a gentle fire, till it is evaporated to dryness.*

17. The principal use of Aloes is as a purgative, in doses of from three to six grains. If administered alone, it is apt to cause griping, nausea, etc.; hence, it is generally given in combination with aromatics, &c. It is ill adapted for children, for persons subject to piles, and for pregnant females.

18. Few medicines are more generally useful for women when suffering from *an Irregular or Suspended state of the Menstrual Discharge;* but it should not be given during pregnancy, nor whilst the menstrual discharge is present. In these cases, especially when the

* Aloes of very good quality may also be prepared from two indigenous species of Aloe, A. Indica, *Royle*, and A. litoralis, *König;* the former inhabiting dry sandy plains in the North-western Provinces, and the latter similar localities on the sea-coasts of the Madras peninsula. The viscid juice with which the thick leaves abound should be collected and evaporated to dryness by exposure in open pans in the sun or over a gentle fire.

patient is pale, thin, and weak, it is best given as follows: Take purified Aloes and Sulphate of Iron, of each, finely powdered, 24 grains; Cinnamon in powder, 60 grains; Honey, sufficient to make a mass; be careful that all the ingredients are well mixed; and divide into 24 pills, of which two are to be taken twice daily.

19. The following is another very good combination:—Take Aloes and Assafœtida, of each 20 grains; beat into a mass with honey, and divide into 12 pills, of which one may be taken twice daily. These pills often prove of great service to women subject to *Hysterical fits*, and *Flatulent distension of the Abdomen*, especially when at the same time there is *Constipation of the Bowels. In Headaches arising from the sudden stoppage either of menstrual discharge or of long-standing bleeding from piles*, these pills often prove useful. Aloes should not be given to persons subject to piles, as they are apt to aggravate the disease.

20. *In cases of Habitual Constipation of the Bowels* great benefit has been found from the persevering use of the following pills:—Take of purified Aloes, 18 grains; Sulphate of Iron, 30 grains; beat into a mass with a little honey, and divide into 24 pills. Of these, one may be taken three times a-day, immediately after the principal meals, till they begin to act upon the bowels gently and then the number may be reduced to two daily. At the end of a week or two another pill may be omitted, and within a month a single pill once or twice a-week will suffice. If at any time they should act powerfully on the bowels as a purgative, they should be discontinued for a time.

21. Alum.

Phitkarí (*Hind.*), Phitkarí (*Beng.*), Fatkarí (*Punj.*), Fatkar, Phatkar (*Kash.*), Pati-káram (*Tam.*, *Tel.*), Chinik-káram (*Mal.*), Pati-kárá (*Can.*), Patikár, Turatí (*Mah.*), Sina-karam (*Cing.*), Keo-khin (*Burm.*), Twas (*Malay*).

22. Alum of good quality is generally procurable in all bazaars. It should be in colourless, transparent, crystalline masses, or pieces of various sizes, with an acid, sweetish, astringent taste. When mixed with impurities, as it often is, it may be rendered fit for medicinal purposes by dissolving it in boiling water, straining the solution, and evaporating it so as to obtain crystals, which should be preserved for use. Alum, whether applied externally or given internally, is a valuable astringent. Dose, from 10 to 20 grains for adults.

23. In that form of *Ophthalmia* commonly known in India by the name of *Country Sore Eyes*, especially when it attacks children, a solution of Alum is often of great service. For children the strength of three grains to an ounce of water is sufficient; but for adults, a solution of double this strength may be used; the eyes should be freely washed with it four or five times a-day, or a cloth wet with it may be kept constantly applied. If the eyelids are much swollen, especially in the morning, they should be well bathed with warm milk, the eyelids should then be carefully separated, and the Alum lotion dropped in. There is a native plan of treatment of these cases

which proves in many instances effectual, but it has the disadvantage of being very painful for a short time. It is as follows:—Place some finely-powdered alum on a heated plate of iron, and whilst it is in a state of fusion add a small portion of lemon or lime-juice, until it forms a black, soft mass. This, whilst hot, is applied entirely round the orbit, care being taken that none of it gets beneath the eyelids, as it causes under such circumstances intense agony. One or two applications, each being allowed to remain on for twelve hours, suffice ordinarily to effect a cure.

24. *After severe Blows on the Eye*, when the pain and heat have subsided, and much discoloration and swelling remain, an ALUM POULTICE is an effectual application. It is made by rubbing up 30 grains of powdered alum with the white of an egg till it forms a coagulum. This placed between two pieces of thin rag or muslin, should be kept applied to the eye for some hours.

25. *In Hæmorrhage from the Lungs, Stomach, Kidneys, Uterus, and other Internal Organs*, Alum, in doses of 10 to 12 grains, thrice daily, with or without opium, may often be given with advantage. It is, however, inadmissible if much fever is present, and should at once be discontinued if after the first few doses the symptoms are at all aggravated. The following, called ALUM WHEY, is a good form of administration:—Boil for ten minutes two drachms of powdered Alum in a pint of milk, and strain; of this, the dose is one and a half to two ounces thrice daily.

This may also be given with the view of checking *Excessive Menstrual Discharges* (*Menorrhagia*) and *Bleeding from Piles.* In this last case, clothes saturated with a solution of Alum in decoction of Galls (145) or Babúl bark (9), in the proportion of two drachms to eight ounces, should be kept constantly applied externally. This application also proves useful in *Prolapsus* (*descent*) *of the Anus*, especially in children. *In Profuse Bleeding from the Nose* injections of a solution of Alum (20 grains to one ounce of water) into the nostril is sometimes effectual; care, however, is required in its use. Powdered Alum, or a very strong saturated solution, applied locally on a compress, occasionally suffices to arrest *Bleeding from Leech-bites, Cuts,* &c.

26. *In the Chronic Diarrhœa of Natives*, the following mixture has been found useful:—Take of Alum ten grains, infusion of Acorus root (12), one and half ounce, Laudanum, five drops; repeat three or four times daily. *In the Diarrhœa which precedes Cholera, and in the early stages of Cholera*, the following powders are worthy of a trial. Take Alum, Catechu, and Cinnamon, of each, powdered, ten grains, mix with honey, and give at a dose. It may be repeated every one or two hours, according to circumstances. It proves useful also in controlling the *Diarrhœa of Phthisis.*

27. As a palliative in *Diabetes*, 'Alum Whey,' prepared as directed in paragraph 25, may be tried; under its use the quantity of urine voided is, in some instances, diminished. *In Albuminuria*, also, it has

been useful in some instances in reducing the proportion of albumen in the urine.

28. *In Hooping Cough*, when the first or acute stage has passed, no remedy is more generally efficacious than Alum, in doses of three or four grains, every four or six hours for a child from two to three years old. It may be given in the form of powder or in solution (Alum 25 grains, Omum Water three ounces) in doses of a dessert-spoonful every four or six hours for a child from two to four years old.

29. *For Relaxed or Ulcerated Sore Throat, for Ulceration and Sponginess of the Gums, in Salivation, and in Fissures of the Tongue in Consumption*, a very useful gargle or mouth wash, is made by dissolving two drachms of Alum in a pint of the decoction of Galls (145) or Babúl Bark (9), and sweetening with honey. *For the small white Ulcers (Aphthæ, or Thrush) in the mouths of infants and young children*, a better application is 20 grains of finely-powdered Alum, incorporated with one ounce of honey. This may be applied twice daily, with the tip of the finger. *In the severer Ulcerative forms of the disease (Ulcerative Stomatitis)* Alum in fine powder, or in strong solution, proves a more effectual application.

30. There is a disease often confounded with *Gonorrhœa*, where the discharge does not come, as it does in true gonorrhœa, from the urethra, but from a sore or excoriated surface between the prepuce and the head of the penis. For this there is no better application than a solution of Alum, 20 grains in one ounce of water. It may be used twice or thrice daily. The

strictest cleanliness should be enforced at the same time. *In Gleet,* a solution of Alum (three grains), in water (one ounce), used, as an injection, twice daily, is often productive of benefit. *In Leucorrhœa and other Vaginal Discharges,* injections of Alum in decoction of Galls or Babúl bark, as advised in the last paragraph, often prove very useful.

31. *In old Chronic spreading and gangrenous Ulcers* so common amongst natives, the following forms an excellent application :—Finely powdered Alum, four drachms; finely powdered Catechu, one drachm; Opium, half a drachm; Ceromel (167), or Kokum butter, or Ghee, one ounce. First, rub down the opium with the ceromel till thoroughly mixed, and then incorporate the other ingredients. A portion of this, spread on soft rag, should be applied to the ulcer night and morning. If it occasion much pain, the proportion of ceromel should be increased. *For Bed-Sores or where these are likely to occur,* Dr. Aitchison describes as an excellent remedy,— a mixture of 30 grains of burnt alum, and the white of a egg. It should be well painted over the part.

32. *For Enlargement of the Joints, especially that of the Knee, and for other Swellings resulting from Blows, Bruises, or Sprains,* the following lotion has been found useful:—Alum, four drachms, Vinegar and Arrack, of each a pint; dissolve, and keep cloths wet with this lotion constantly to the affected part. *In Scorpion Bites,* Alum moistened with water and locally applied often affords instantaneous relief (Dr. Saunders).

33. **Assafœtida.**

Hing (*Hind.*, *Duk.*, *Beng.*, *Punj.*, *Mah.*, *Guz.*), Yang (*Kash.*), Káyam, Perun-gáyam (*Tam.*), Inguva (*Tel.*), Perun-gáyam, Káyam (*Mal.*), Perun-káyam (*Cing.*), Shinkhu or Shingu (*Burm.*), Hingu (*Malay*).

34. Assafœtida of good quality may be obtained in most bazaars. The moister and most strongly smelling kinds should be chosen for medical purposes. It may be given in the form of pill, in doses of from five to ten grains; or in that of mixture, prepared by rubbing down in a mortar five drachms of Assafœtida in a pint of hot water, and straining, and setting aside to cool. Of this solution, which is thick and milky, the dose is from one to two tablespoonsfuls. Its nauseous taste is a great objection to its use.

35. *In Hysterical Fits* and in *Fainting, Nervous Palpitations, and other affections connected with Hysteria*, Assafœtida proves most useful. When the symptoms are urgent, as in fits, &c., it is best given in the liquid form (*ante*), but where the object is rather to combat the tendency to this state, and to make an impression on the system, the solid form should be preferred. For this purpose it may be advantageously combined with aloes, as advised in Sect. 19.

36. *In Flatulence, Flatulent Colic, and Spasmodic Affections of the Bowels*, especially when connected with hysteria, it is best given in the form of enema (30 grains in four ounces of water); but if this is not practicable, it may be given by mouth in the liquid

form advised above. A teaspoonful of the mixture, with a little Omum water, is often very effectual in relieving the *Flatulent Colic of Children.* It may also be tried in the *Convulsions of pale weakly children.* An Assafœtida enema is an effectual means of removing *Thread worms* from the rectum and lower bowel.

37. *In the obstinate Coughs of Childhood,* remaining after attacks of inflammation, and also *the advanced stages of Hooping Cough,* the mixture has also occasionally been found of great service in doses of a teaspoonful four or five times daily. It has also been recommended in the *Chronic Bronchitis and Asthma of Adults;* its disagreeable smell and taste is a great bar to its use, but this may, in a great measure, be obviated by giving it in the form of pill.

38. **Asteracantha (Barleria) longifolia,** *Nees.*

Talmakháné, Gokshura (*Hind.*), Kolsí (*Duk.*), Kánta-koliká (*Beng.*), Tálmakhánáh (*Punj.*, *Kash.*), Nir-mulli (*Tam.*), Niru-gobbi (*Tel.*), Vayal-chulli (*Mal.*), Kolava-like (*Can.*), Tál-makháná (*Mah.*), Ikkiri (*Cing.*), Súpadán (*Burm.*).

39. The whole of this plant, common in moist sites throughout India, but especially the root, which in the dried state is sold in the bazaars, enjoys a high repute amongst the natives as a diuretic in *Dropsical cases,* which European experience has, in a great measure, tended to confirm. It may be given in the form of decoction, prepared by boiling one ounce of the root in a pint of water for ten minutes, straining,

and taking the whole in divided doses during the day. The following is advised by Baboo Kanny Lall Dey :—Take of freshly-dried Asteracantha leaves, two ounces; Distilled Vinegar, 16 ounces; macerate for three days; press and strain. Of this, the dose is from one to three tablespoonfuls in water thrice daily.

40. **Atis, or Atees.** The root of Aconitum heterophyllum, *Wallich.*

Atís (*Hind.*), Atviká (*Duk.*), Atis, Batis, Patis (*Punj.*), Mohand-i-guj-saféd, Hong-i-saféd (*Kash.*), Ati-vadayam (*Tam.*), Ati-vasa (*Tel.*).

41. Atís, as met with in the bazaars, occurs in the form of small tuberous roots, tapering towards a point, from one to one and a half inches, or more in length, and from three-eighths to a quarter of an inch in thickness; grey externally, slightly wrinkled longitudinally, and marked here and there with rootlet scars, easily friable; internally white, farinaceous, inodorous, and of a pure bitter taste, devoid of acidity or astringency. This last character serves to distinguish it from all other roots sold under the same name. *Every root should be broken across, and all which are not pure white, with a short, starchy fracture and pure bitter taste, should be discarded.* Further, if on chewing a small piece, it cause a feeling of tingling or peculiar sensation on the tongue, followed by even the smallest degree of numbness or altered sensation, it should on no account be used. Mr. Boughton discovered in it an alkaloid to which he gave the name of *Atisine.*

42. The chief use of Atís is in the treatment of *Intermittent Fever and other periodical fevers,* and in these it often proves most valuable. It should be given in doses of half a drachm (30 grains), mixed with a little water, every four or six hours during the intermissions, commencing its use during or towards the close of the sweating stage. For children the dose may be reduced one-half, or three-fourths, according to age. For combating the *Debility after Fevers and other diseases,* Atís is an excellent tonic, in doses of five to ten grains thrice daily.

43. **Bael Fruit.** The fruit of Ægle Marmelos, *Corr.*

Bél, Si-phal (*Hind., Beng., Punj.*), Bél-phal (*Duk.*), Vilva or Bilva-pazham (*Tam.*), Bilva-pandu, Márédu-pandu (*Tel.*), Kúvalap-pazham (*Mal.*), Bilapatri-hannu (*Can.*), Bél-phal (*Guz.*), Béláchaphala, Bela (*Mah.*), Bélli, Bélli-ka (*Cing.*), Ushi-si, Ushi-ti (*Burm.*), Buah Bail (*Malay*).

44. The half-ripe fruit is best suited for medical use, and that freshly gathered is preferable to that which has been kept a long time, as is generally the case with the bazaar article.* European experience

* In bazaar specimens, the Wood-apple (fruit of Feronia Elephantum) is often substituted for Bael. Though they bear a close resemblance externally, they can easily be distinguished by opening them. In the true Bael, there are, in the centre of the pulp, a number of cells, from five to eighteen, each containing one or more seeds and glutinous mucus, whilst in the Wood-apple there are no cells, and the seeds are embedded in the pulp.

has confirmed the native opinion that it is a remedy of much value in cases of *obstinate Diarrhœa and Dysentery* when unattended by fever, and the patient is weak and dyspeptic. It proves especially serviceable when any signs of *Scurvy* are present. It is best given as follows :—Take of the soft gummy fluid from the interior of the fruit two ounces, mix this with three or four ounces of water, sweeten to taste, and, if procurable, add a lump of ice. This draught should be repeated twice or thrice daily. *In the obstinate Diarrhœa and Dysentery of Children*, it may safely be given in doses of from one quarter to one half the above quantity, according to age. The Fluid Extract of the *dried* Bael is regarded by many as superior to any other preparations of this fruit. The dose is from half a drachm to a drachm, twice or thrice daily for an adult. Dietetic Bael is also a valuable preparation.*

45. *In Irregularity of the Bowels, presenting alternations of Diarrhœa and Constipation*, one draught, as described in the last section, taken in the early

* Dr. Aitchison suggests that a supply of DIETETIC BAEL (prepared by Messrs. Bathgate & Co., of Calcutta) should be kept in store. 'It consists,' he remarks, 'of the pulp of dried Bael fruit carefully pulverised and mixed with a certain proportion of arrowroot. It is an excellent preparation to be used in those cases when Bael is prescribed, and where the fresh fruit cannot be got of good quality, *e. g.* the Bael fruit grown in the Punjab is not to be compared with that of the more moist and tropical regions. Besides using this in actual disease it makes a good substitute in a patient's diet owing to its pleasant aromatic flavour.'

morning, often exercises a most beneficial effect in regulating the bowels. Where much debility exists, and the stomach is weak and irritable, it is apt to disagree, occasioning eructations, &c., in which case it may be tried in smaller doses, or be given at bed-time in place of early morning.

46. **Betel or Betle Leaves.** The fresh leaves of Chavica (Piper) Betle, *Retz.*

Pán (*Hind.*, *Duk.*, *Beng.*, *Punj.*, and *Guz.*), Vettilai (*Tam.*) Tamala-páku, Nága-valli (*Tel.*), Vetrila (*Mal.*), Viledele (*Can.*), Videchapána (*Mah.*), Balát (*Cing.*), Kún-yoe (*Burm.*), Seereh (*Malay*).

47. These leaves are in almost universal use amongst the natives of India as a masticatory, in conjunction with lime and areca-nut. There are two ways in which they may be usefully employed medicinally:—

48. *In Coughs, especially those of Infancy and Childhood, where there is difficulty of breathing*, the application of betel leaves, warmed, smeared with oil, and applied in layers over the chest, often affords speedy and marked relief. It is a native practice, the utility of which has been confirmed by European experience. It can do no harm, may do much good, and is therefore worthy of a trial in all cases. The same application has been recommended in *Congestion and other affections of the Liver.*

49. For the purpose of *Arresting the Secretion of Milk*, when from any cause this may be desirable,

betel leaves, warmed by the fire, and placed in layers over the breasts, are stated to be very effectual. Thus employed they are also said to be useful in reducing *Glandular Swellings.*

50. **Bonduc Nut.** The fruit of Cæsalpinia (Guilandina) Bonducella, *Linn.*

Kat-kalijá, Kat-karanj (*Hind.*), Gajgá (*Duk.*), Ṇátá, Nátú-koranjá (*Beng.*), Kanjúá (*Punj.*), Kazhar-shik-káy (*Tam.*), Gech-chak-káya (*Tel.*), Kalanchik-kuru (*Mal.*), Gajaga-káyi (*Can.*), Gajaga (*Mah.*), Gájgá (*Guz.*), Kumbura-atta (*Cing.*), Kalén-zi (*Burm.*), Buah gorah (*Malay*).

51. These nuts, common in all the bazaars of India, are roundish or ovoid in shape, about half an inch, or more, in diameter, smooth, hard, of a grey or leaden colour externally, contain a white starchy kernel of a pure bitter taste. Their efficacy appears to reside in a bitter oil. Mr. Broughton failed to detect in them any special crystalline principle.

52. *In Intermittent Fevers,* especially in those of the natives, this remedy has been found very useful. It is adapted only for mild, uncomplicated cases, and is best given in the following form:—Take of Bonduc seeds, deprived of their shells and powdered, one ounce; Black Pepper powdered one ounce; mix thoroughly, and keep in a well-stoppered bottle. Of this the dose is from 15 to 30 grains three times a day for adults. In smaller doses it is a good tonic in *Debility after Fevers and other diseases.* The bark of

the root of the Bonduc shrub in 10 grain doses is reported to be even more effectual in the above cases than the seeds themselves.

53. **Borax.** Biborate of Soda.

Sohágá, Tinkál (*Hind.*), Sohágá (*Beng.*, *Duk.*, *Punj.*), Vávut, Váwuth (*Kash.*), Venkáram (*Tam.*), Elegáram (*Tel.*), Ponkáram, Vellakaram (*Mal.*), Biligára (*Can.*), Vengáram, Puskara (*Cing.*), Lakhiya, Let-khya (*Burm.*), Pijar (*Malay*).

54. Borax of good quality is met with in most bazaars; if good it should be in transparent, colourless, crystalline masses or pieces of various sizes, inodorous, with a cool saltish taste. After having been exposed to the air for some time, as that found in the bazaars has generally been, it becomes covered with a whitish powder or efflorescence, which being removed shows the transparent crystal beneath. If brown or dirty, or otherwise impure, it may be rendered fit for medical use by dissolving one pound of it with one drachm of quicklime in three pints of water, straining through cloth and evaporating by exposure to the sun in an open vessel or over a gentle fire. Dose from 20 to 40 grains for an adult.

55. *In Aphthæ or Thrush* (small white spots and ulcerations in the mouths of infants and young children) a mixture of powdered Borax (1 drachm) and Honey (1 ounce) is one of the best applications which can be used; it should be applied by means of the finger to the spot twice or thrice daily. *In Fissures*

or Cracks in the Tongue in adults, which occur in the advanced stages of Consumption, Fever, &c., an application twice the strength of the above, proves highly serviceable. *In Mercurial Salivation*, a solution of Borax (half an ounce), in water (eight ounces) forms an excellent gargle.

56. *To Sore Nipples* a solution of Borax, one drachm to one ounce of water, should be applied before and after suckling the infant, or it may be employed in the form of ointment (a drachm of Borax to an ounce of ghee). These applications are also serviceable when applied to *inflamed and painful Piles.*

57. *As a means of allaying the distressing Irritation of the Genital Organs, both of males and females*, the latter especially, a solution of Borax (half an ounce) in eight ounces of water or Camphor julep (67) sometimes affords more relief than anything else. Cloths saturated with it should be kept to the parts, and in the case of women it should also be used in the form of vaginal injection. It also proves very useful in allaying the *Irritation of Nettle-rash, Prickly Heat, and other Skin Diseases.*

58. *In prolonged and tedious Labours* dependent apparently on want of action or power in the uterus to expel the fœtus, and in *Abortion* under the same circumstances, 30 grains of Borax with 10 grains of powdered Cinnamon, in a little warm conjee, may be given every one or two hours to the extent of three or four doses. This may also be given in *Convulsions attendant on Labours.* In doses of 10 grains, 10 with of Cinnamon, thrice daily, it also occasionally proves

useful in *Suspension or Irregularity of the Menstrual Discharge* and in some *Chronic Uterine Affections.*

59. *To Ulcerated Buboes, and Sloughing Ulcers*, a solution of Borax (two drachms in a pint of water or Camphor julep) often proves very useful by cleansing the surface and hastening the healing process. It should be applied on rags well over the whole sore, and renewed frequently by night and day. For dressing *Delhi Sores*, and stimulating them to healthy action, a favourite application is composed of Borax, Sulphur, and Catechu, of each finely powdered, one drachm, and lard or ghee one ounce. This may be advantageously used in other forms of *Ulceration.*

60. *For Ringworm*, a solution of Borax (one drachm) in distilled vinegar (two ounces) is stated to be an effectual application.

61. **Butea Gum. Bengal Kino.** The inspissated juice obtained from the stems of Butea frondosa, *Roxb.**

Palás-kí-gond (*Hind.*, *Duk.*), Pálásh-gun (*Beng.*), Dhák-kí-gond (*Punj.*), Kamar-kash (*Kash.*), Muruk-kan-pishin, Palásha-pishin (*Tam.*), Palásha-banka, Móduga-banka (*Tel.*), Plách-cha-pasha (*Mal.*), Muttaga-góndu (*Can.*), Phalása-cha-gónda (*Mah.*), Khákar-nu-gún (*Guz.*), Káliya-melliyam (*Cing.*), Páv-si (*Burm.*).

* Pterocarpus Marsupium, *D. C.*, which yields the officinal Kino, inhabits the forests of Ceylon and the Indian Peninsula as far north as Behar; but almost all, if not the whole, of the Kino met with in bazaars is the produce of Butea frondosa or B. superba; but this is a matter of little moment, as it appears to be equally effectual as an astringent.

62. Butea Gum occurs in the form of irregular shining fragments, seldom as large as a pea, more or less mixed with adherent pieces of greyish bark, of an intense ruby colour and astringent taste. Its astringency is due to the presence of tannic and gallic acids. It is an excellent astringent, similar to Catechu, but, being milder in operation, it is better adapted for children and delicate females. The dose of the powdered gum is 10 to 30 grains, with a few grains of powdered Cinnamon. It may be used with advantage in *Chronic Diarrhœa, Pyrosis (Water brash), and in those forms of Dyspepsia attended with increased secretion.* In these cases the addition of a small portion of opium increases its efficacy.

63. **Butea Seeds.** The seeds of Butea frondosa, *Roxb.*

Palás-ké-bínj (*Hind.*), Palás-páprá (*Duk., Beng.*), Dhák-papri, Palás-páprí (*Punj.*), Khálás-pápúr (*Kash.*), Porasum-virai, Murukkam-virai (*Tam.*), Palásha-vittulu, Moduga-vittulu (*Tel.*), Pláshu, Murukka-vitta (*Mal.*), Muttaga-bíjá (*Can.*), Phalásá-cha-bí (*Mah.*), Palás-páparo (*Guz.*), Kaliya-atta (*Cing.*), Páv-si (*Burm.*).

64. Butea seeds are thin, flat, oval, or kidney-shaped, of a mahogany brown colour, $1\frac{1}{4}$ to $1\frac{3}{4}$ inches in length, almost devoid of taste and smell. European experience has confirmed the high opinion held by the Mohammedan doctors as to their power in *expelling Lumbrici, or Round Worm,* so common

amongst the natives of India. The seeds should be first soaked in water, and the testa, or shell, carefully removed, the kernel should then be dried and reduced to powder. Of this the dose is 20 grains thrice daily for three successive days, followed on the fourth day by a dose of Castor Oil. Under the use of this remedy, thus administered in the practice of Dr. Oswald, 125 lumbrici in one instance, and between 70 and 80 in another, were expelled. It has the disadvantage of occasionally purging when its vermifuge properties are not apparent; in some instances also it has been found to excite vomiting and to irritate the kidneys: and though these ill effects do not ordinarily follow, yet they indicate caution in its employment.

65. *For destroying Maggots in Unhealthy Ulcers*, so commonly met with amongst the natives, Raghupatie Mohun Rao (*Indian Medical Gazette*, Dec. 2, 1879, p. 346) directs the powder of these seeds to be sprinkled over the surface to kill them.

66. **Camphor.**

Káfúr (*Hind.*, *Punj.*), Káphúr (*Beng.*), Karruppúram *or* Karppúram (*Tam.*), Karpúram (*Tel.*, *Mal.*), Karpúra (*Can.*), Kapúra (*Mah.*), Kapúr, Karpúr (*Guz.*), Kapuru (*Cing.*), Payo, Piyo (*Burm.*), Kapor baroos (*Malay*).

Several varieties of Camphor are met with in the bazaars. That best suited for medicinal use should be in masses or lumps, white, translucent, of a crystalline structure, of a powerful penetrating odour, and pungent taste. Much of the camphor sold in the bazaars is worthless. Dose, from two to five grains or more for an adult.

67. Camphor Water, or Julep, as it is commonly called, may always be advantageously kept ready prepared for domestic use; it is made by adding two drachms of Camphor to a quart bottle of water, and setting aside for a few days. Of this the dose for an adult is about a wine-glassful. It is a good vehicle for other medicines.

68. Camphor Liniment is formed by dissolving one ounce of Camphor in four ounces of Cocoa-nut, Sesamum, or other bland oil. It is an excellent application in *Chronic Rheumatism, Lumbago, Enlargement of the Joints, Glandular Swellings, Bruises, Sprains, Muscular Pain, especially that of the loins to which women are subject during Pregnancy and the Menstrual periods*, and other cases attended with local pain. It should be well rubbed in night and morning for 10 or 15 minutes; friction in these cases playing an important part.

69. *In Chronic Rheumatism*, in addition to its use externally, as advised in the last paragraph, it may be given internally in a dose of five grains with one grain of Opium at bed time; it affords relief by causing copious perspiration, which should be promoted by a draught of infusion of Ginger (154) and by additional bed clothes. An excellent vapour bath for these cases may be made by substituting half an ounce of Camphor placed on a heated plate for the chattie of hot

water described in Section 397. Thus employed, it causes speedy and copious perspiration. Care, however, is necessary to prevent the patient inhaling the vapour, which is of comparatively little consequence when simple water is being employed.

70. *In Asthma,* Camphor in four grain doses, with an equal quantity of Assafœtida, in the form of pill, repeated every second or third hour during a paroxysm, affords in some instances great relief. Turpentine stupes (362) to the chest should be used at the same time. Many cases of *Difficulty of Breathing* are relieved by the same means. These pills also sometimes relieve violent *Palpitation of the Heart. In the Coughs of Childhood,* Camphor Liniment (68), previously warmed, well rubbed in over the chest at nights, often exercises a beneficial effect. For young children, the strength of the liniment should be reduced one half or more by the addition of some bland oil.

71. *In Rheumatic and Nervous Headaches,* a very useful application is one ounce of Camphor dissolved in a pint of vinegar, and then diluted with one or two parts of water. Cloths saturated with it should be kept constantly to the part.

72. *In Spermatorrhœa, and in all involuntary Seminal discharges,* few medicines are more generally useful than Camphor in doses of four grains with half-a-grain of Opium, taken each night at bed time. *In Gonorrhœa,* to relieve that painful symptom, *Chordee,* the same prescription is generally very effectual; but it may be necessary to increase the quantity of Opium to one grain, and it is advisable to apply the Camphor

Liniment (68) along the under surface of the penis as far back as the anus. *To relieve that distressing Irritation of the Generative Organs which some women suffer from so severely,* it will be found that five or six grains of Camphor taken in the form of pill twice or three times daily, according to the severity of the symptoms, will sometimes afford great relief. In each of these cases, it is important to keep the bowels freely open.

73. *In painful Affections of the Uterus,* Camphor in six or eight grain doses often affords much relief. The Liniment (68) should at the same time be well rubbed into the loins. *In the Convulsions attendant on Childbirth,* the following pills may be tried :—Camphor and Calomel, of each five grains. Beat into a mass with a little honey, and divide into two pills ; to be followed an hour subsequently by a full dose of castor oil or other purgative.

74. *In the advanced stages of Fever, Small Pox,* and *Measles,* when the patient is low, weak, and exhausted, and when there are at the same time delirium, muttering, and sleeplessness, three grains of Camphor with an equal quantity of Assafœtida, may be given even every third hour ; Turpentine stupes (362) or Mustard poultices (247) being applied at the same time to the feet or over the region of the heart. It should be discontinued if it causes headache or increased heat of the scalp. Its use requires much discrimination and caution.

75. *To prevent Bed Sores,* it is advisable to make a strong solution of Camphor in arrack or brandy, and with this night and morning to bathe, for a few minutes,

the parts which from continued pressure are likely to become affected. *Gangrenous or Sloughing Ulcerations* often sensibly improve, and heal under the local application of powdered Camphor.

76. **Capsicum.** The ripe dried fruit of Capsicum fastigiatum, *Blume.*

Lál-mirch, Gách-mirch (*Hind.*), Mirchí, Lál-mirchí (*Duk*), Lal-morich, Lanká-morich (*Beng.*), Lal-mirch (*Punj.*), Mirch-wángun (*Kash.*), Mulagáy, Milagáy (*Tam.*), Mirapa-káya (*Tel.*), Kappal-melaka (*Mal.*), Ménashiná-káyi (*Can.*), Mir-singá (*Mah.*), Lál-mirich, Marchu (*Guz.*), Miris (*Cing.*), Náyu-si (*Burm.*), Chalie, Loda-cheena (*Malay*).

77. A powerful stimulant; the bruised fruit applied locally in the form of poultice acts energetically as a rubefacient, and, added to Mustard poultices, greatly increases their activity. In the absence of mustard, Capsicum poultices may be substituted, but, being more energetic in operation, require more care; if left on too long they will cause blisters.

78. *In Scarlatina,* the following mixture has attained much repute in the West Indies. Take two table spoonfuls of bruised Capsicum and two tea spoonfuls of Salt; beat them into a paste, and add half a pint of boiling Water; when cold, strain, and add half a pint of Vinegar. Dose for an adult, one table spoonful every four hours; to be diminished for children according to age, or the severity of the attack. The same formula forms an excellent gargle in the

Sore Throat which accompanies this disease, as well as in ordinary *Relaxed Sore Throat, Hoarseness,* &c.

79. Capsicum is a very useful adjunct to Aloes and other remedies for *Dyspepsia, Loss of Appetite,* &c. *In Diarrhœa, arising fvom the use of putrid food, especially fish,* Capsicum in five grain doses in the form of pill has been found most useful.

80. **Cassia alata,** *Linn.* Ringworm Shrub.

Dádmurdan, Dád-ká-pát (*Hind.*), Dádmurdan, Dádmari (*Beng.*), Dát-ká-pattá, Viláyatí-agtí (*Duk.*), Ponwar (*Punj.*), Shimai-agatti, Vandu-kolli (*Tam.*), Shíma-avishi-chettu (*Tel.*), Shima-akatti (*Mal.*), Shíme-agase (*Can.*), Attóra (*Cing.*), Timbó-mezali, Mezali-gi (*Burm.*).

81. This handsome shrub, with its large conspicuous spike of yellow flowers, is common in gardens and waste places throughout India. Its leaves have attained a well-earned repute as a local remedy in *Skin Diseases,* especially in *Ringworm;* hence one of its common English names of *Ringworm Bush or Shrub.* The ordinary form of application is a sort of ointment made by bruising the fresh leaves with Sesamum, Cocoa-nut, or other bland oil; but a far better preparation is made by bruising the fresh leaves, with lemon or lime juice, into a thick paste. Whichever preparation is employed, it should be thoroughly well rubbed in over the affected part twice daily till a cure is effected. The more recent the case the greater will be the prospect of a speedy cure. Long-standing chronic cases often resist its influence.

82. **Castor Oil.**—The expressed oil of the seeds of Ricinus communis, *Linn.*

Arandí-ká-tél (*Hind.*, *Punj.*), Yarandí-ká-tél (*Duk.*), Bhérandá-tail (*Beng.*), A'manak-kenney (*Tam.*), A'mudam (*Tel.*), Kottenná (*Mal.*), Haralenne (*Can.*), Eran-déla (*Mah.*), Dívás, Yerandi-nu-tél (*Guz.*), Endaru-tel (*Cing.*), Kesu-si (*Burm.*), Miniak jarak (*Malay*).

83. Castor Oil, of various degrees of purity, is met with in most bazaars. The dark brown viscid oil (obtained by boiling, and subsequent expression of the seeds) should be avoided, on account of its acridity. The best kind is clear, of a pale straw colour, and with a slightly nauseous taste. The 'cold-drawn expressed oil' should always be used when procurable, as it generally is in most large bazaars. It is an excellent purgative when the object is simply to clear out the bowels. It is especially adapted for children and for women after confinements. The ordinary dose for a child is about a tea spoonful, but it may be gradually raised according to the age of the patient, to two table spoonfuls (one ounce), which is the full dose for an adult. It is best given floating on milk, strong coffee, or Omum water. *In painful affections of the Rectum* Castor Oil in small doses is often of great service, softening the fæces and lubricating the passages without weakening the patient. (*Mr. Curling.*) The same remark applies to *Piles,* or when it is desirable to prevent the patient straining at stool, but, as a general rule, it is inferior to Sulphur, *q. v.*

84. *For Sore Nipples* nothing, according to Dr. Conant Foster (*Practitioner*, April 1872), is so beneficial as Castor Oil. The nipple should be smeared freely with it each time the child is removed from the breast. Rags or lint are unnecessary and injurious.

85. **The leaves of the Castor Oil plant** deserve notice *as a means of increasing the secretion of Milk.* For this purpose a decoction is made by boiling a large handful of the plant in six or eight pints of water. With this the breasts are bathed for a quarter of an hour, and then the boiled leaves, in the form of a poultice, spread over them. In a few hours the effects of the application are manifest. A simpler mode of application, said to be equally effectual, consists in applying layers of the fresh leaves, simply warmed before a fire, over the breasts.

86. **Catechu.** An extract from the heart-wood of Acacia Catechu, *Willd.*

Kát, Kath (*Hind.*, *Punj.*), Kát (*Beng.*), Kathah (*Duk.*), Khaīrah, Kuth (*Kash.*), Káshu, Kátta-kámbu (*Tam.*), Kánchu (*Tel.*), Kátta (*Mal.*), Káchu (*Can.*), Kath-tho (*Guz.*), Kaipu (*Cing.*), Sházi (*Burm.*), Gambir or Kachu (*Malay*).

87. Several varieties of Catechu are met with in the bazaars. That best adapted for medical use occurs in the form of masses consisting of layers, occasionally enveloped in rough leaves of a blackish brown colour, easily fractured, of a very astringent taste.

88. *In Diarrhœa unattended by fever* Catechu is of much value; ten or fifteen grains in powder, with an equal quantity of powdered Cinnamon, may be given in honey or jaggery three or four times a day if necessary; or it may be given in infusion prepared by macerating three drachms of bruised Catechu, and one drachm of bruised Cinnamon in a half-pint of boiling water for two hours, and straining. Dose from one and a half to two ounces thrice daily. From five to ten drops of Laudanum to each dose add to its efficacy, or one grain of Opium may be given at bed-time. These doses are suited only for adults; for *the Diarrhœa of Children,* three or four grains finely powdered Catechu, with an equal quantity of powdered Cinnamon, generally answer well.

89. *In Mercurial Salivation, in Ulceration and Sponginess of the Gums,* a small piece of Catechu allowed slowly to dissolve in the mouth is often of great service. The same measure is often useful in *Relaxed Sore Throat, Hoarseness, Loss of Voice,* &c. *In Toothache,* where there is a decayed tooth, with a piece of loose flesh growing within, great relief sometimes results from inserting into the hollow a small piece of Catechu, and retaining it there till it is dissolved.

90. *Chronic Ulcerations, attended by much or fœtid discharge,* often speedily improve under the use of an ointment composed of a drachm of finely powdered Catechu and an ounce of Lard or Ceromel (167). In obstinate cases the addition of sixteen grains of finely-powdered Sulphate of Copper to the above greatly

increases its efficacy. Another mode of treating these old ulcers is bathing them twice or thrice daily with an infusion of Catechu (six drachms to a pint of water), and dressing in the intervals with Ceromel. The above infusion proves effectual in some instances as a preventative of *Sore Nipples,* for which purpose the breasts should be bathed with it daily, for some six weeks prior to the confinement, and thus the tissues become so hardened that when the infant begins to suck any ill effects are obviated.

90 *bis.* **Charcoal Wood, Charcoal.**

Lakrí-ka-kóyelah (*Hind.*), Lakri-ká-kôlsá (*Duk.*), Kásh-tha-kóyalá (*Beng.*), Aduppu-kari (*Tam.*), Katta-boggu (*Tel.*), Atuppa-kari, Muttí-kari (*Mal.*), Kattige-iddallu (*Can.*), Láka-dácha-kólasé (*Mah.*), Lákdu-kôelo (*Guz.*), Thén-misu-e (*Burm.*), Anguru (*Cing.*), Ahrang (*Malay*), Kôiláh (*Punj.*), Tsuíng (*Kash.*).

91. Charcoal is an article of great importance in a sanatory and medical as well as in an economical point of view. It possesses no mean power as a deodorizer, and in close sick rooms the smell of the air is deprived of much of its unpleasantness by hanging about the apartment thin muslin bags loosely filled with roughly powdered charcoal. The charcoal requires to be renewed occasionally. For purifying water an effectual plan is to boil it with a good-sized piece of freshly prepared charcoal; it also forms an excellent filter, placed in alternate layers with river sand, as is in use

by the natives of Southern India. Charcoal, especially that of the Areca or Betel nut, forms an excellent tooth-powder; but it is essential that it should be *very* finely powdered, or it may scratch the enamel of the teeth. Lastly, it is of great value in forming the CHARCOAL POULTICE, which is made by adding finely powdered charcoal to a common Rice poultice (322) in proportion of one part of the former to three of the latter. A little of the Charcoal should also be sprinkled over the surface of the poultice previous to applying it. This is a valuable application to *Ulcers and Wounds attended by a fœtid discharge;* it proves useful in correcting the bad odour and stimulating tó healthy action.

92. **Chaulmugra.*** (The seeds of Gynocardia odorata, *R. Brown.*)

Chaulmúgra or Chál-mogré-ké-bínj (*Hind.*).

93. Chaulmúgra seeds are about an inch in length, of an ovoid form, rendered more or less irregular by mutual compression. The shell, greyish brown, smooth and fragile, contains a large kernel, which by expression yields a fixed oil which has a peculiar and slightly unpleasant smell and taste. The oil procured from the bazaars is usually impure, and hence objectionable for internal administration.

* In Southern India, where Chaulmúgra is rarely obtainable, the oil of the seeds of a tree of the same family, Hydnocarpus inebrians, *Vahl.* (Néradi-muttu, *Tam.*, Niradi-vittulu, *Tel.*) seems well worthy of a trial. This oil has a great repute amongst the natives of Malabar as a remedy in leprosy.

94. *In Leprosy* Chaulmúgra has been used with excellent effect; it has also been advantageously administered in *Scrofula, Skin Diseases, and Chronic Rheumatism.* The dose of the seeds coarsely powdered is about six grains, thrice daily, in the form of pill, gradually increased to three or four times that amount, or until it causes nausea, when the dose should be diminished, or the use of the remedy suspended for a time. This is the best form of administration. The dose of the oil is from five to six drops, gradually increased as in the case of the seeds. During the use of this remedy it is advisable to avoid all salt meats, acids, spices, and sweetmeats; on the other hand, its operation is aided by butter, ghee, and oily articles of diet. It might, perhaps, be advantageously combined with a course of fish-liver oil.

95. An ointment, prepared by beating the seeds, deprived of their shells, into a paste of the requisite consistence, with a little ghee, or simple ointment, has been found of great service as a local application in some *obstinate Skin Diseases.*

96. **Chiretta.** The dried plant Ophelia Chirata, *D.C.*

Charáyatah (*Hind., Duk.*), Shirat-kuch-chi, Nila-vémbu (*Tam.*), Nelá-vému (*Tel.*), Cherota (*Beng.*), Chiraita, Kiraita (*Punj.*), Chiraiet (*Kash.*), Chiráyitá (*Mah.*), Chírayata (*Guz.*), Bincohamba (*Cing.*), Sekhági (*Burm.*), Chrita (*Malay*).

97. Stems about three feet long, of the thickness of a goose-quill, round, smooth, pale-brown, branched, branches opposite ; flowers small, numerous, panicled; the whole plant intensely bitter. These characters belong to the officinal Chiretta, but there are met with, in almost every part of India, numerous varieties which differ more or less from it in many respects, except in bitterness, which pervades them all. They also partake, for the most part, in the same medicinal properties.

98. Chiretta is a good bitter tonic, and renders the practitioner in India independent of imported articles of the same class. It is best given as follows: take Chiretta, bruised one ounce, Hot Water a pint; infuse for six hours or more and strain. Dose from two to three ounces three times daily. A drachm of bruised Cloves or Cinnamon, or Cardamom seeds, increases its efficacy and improves its flavour. It may be given in all cases of *Debility, especially after Fevers, in Indigestion, Loss of Appetite,* &c. It may also be given in mild cases of *Ague or Intermittent Fever ;* but this is spoken of in Art. Galls, *q. v.*

99. A good form of employing Chiretta as a tonic is to add two ounces of the bruised stems to a bottle of Sherry and let it stand for a week. Of this a wine-glassful should be taken once or twice daily, one hour before meals, in *Indigestion, Loss of Appetite,* and other cases mentioned in the last section.

100. **Cinnamon.** The dried bark of Cinnamomum Zeylanicum, *Nees.*

Dár-cíní (*Hind. Punj.*), Dál-chíní (*Duk.*, *Beng.*, *Kash.*, *Guz.*), Lavanga-pattai, Karuvá-pattai (*Tam.*), Lavanga patta (*Mal.*, *Tel.*), Dála-chini (*Can.*, *Mah.*), Kurundo (*Cing.*), Timbo-tik-yobo (*Burm.*), Kulit-manis (*Malay*).

101. The above names belong only to the true Cinnamon, which is procurable in most bazaars; it requires to be distinguished from the country Cinnamon, the bark of Cinnamomum iners (Jangli-dalchiní, *Hind.*, Kattu-karuvá-pattai, *Tam.*), which is very inferior. The former occurs in small closely rolled quills, containing several smaller quills within them of a light yellowish-brown colour, fragrant odour, and warm sweet aromatic taste; the latter is a much larger and thicker bark, generally curved, but seldom completely quilled, the taste less sweet, with some degree of astringency, and the smell less fragrant.

102. Cinnamon is a pleasant aromatic stimulant and carminative, closely allied in medical properties and uses to Cloves (105), for which it may be substituted when the latter are not available. It is an agreeable adjunct to many other medicines.

103. **Cloves.** The dried unexpanded flower-buds of Caryophyllus aromaticus, *Linn.*

Lóng (*Hind.*, *Beng.*), Lavang (*Duk.*), Kirámbu, Ilavangap-pú (*Tam.*), Lavango-pú, Lavangálu (*Tel.*), Karámpu (*Mal.*), Lavanga (*Can.*, *Mah.*), Lavang (*Guz.*), Krábu-nati (*Cing.*), Láũng (*Punj.*), Raung (*Kash.*), Leniah-poén, Lenang-poén (*Burm*), Bunga Chingkeh (*Malay*).

104. The Cloves met with in the bazaars are often old and worthless. Those suited for medical use should have a strong, fragrant odour, a bitter, spicy, pungent taste, and should emit a trace of oil when indented with the nail.

105. Cloves are a good useful stimulant and carminative, stronger than Cinnamon, which, however, may be advantageously substituted when the former are either of inferior quality or not procurable. A pleasant and serviceable mixture is made by infusing three drachms of bruised Cloves in a pint of boiling water, and straining when cold. Of this the dose is from one to two ounces in *Indigestion*, *Flatulence*, *Colic and Spasmodic Affections of the Bowels.* It sometimes succeeds in checking *Vomiting*, *especially that attendant on Pregnancy.* A mixture of equal parts of the infusions of Cloves and Chiretta (98) has often excellent effect in *Debility*, *Loss of Appetite*, and in *Convalescence after Fevers.*

106. **Cocculus Indicus.** The fruits of Anamirta Cocculus, *W. et A.*

Kákmárí-ke-bínj (*Hind.*, *Duk.*), Kàkà-màri (*Beng.*), Kákkáy-kolli-varai, Pén-kottai (*Tam.*), Káka-mári, Káki-champa (*Tel.*), Karanta-kattin-káya, Pollak-káya (*Mal.*), Kaka-mári-bíjá (*Can.*), Tittaval (*Cing.*).

107. The dried fruit, sold in most bazaars, is rather larger than a full-sized pea, somewhat kidney-shaped, blackish brown, wrinkled, containing a yel-

lowish, oily, bitter, kidney-shaped kernel inclosed in a two-valved shell. It is powerfully poisonous and is never administered internally; its sole use, and in this respect it is very effectual, is as an insecticide, *i.e.*, as an agent *for destroying pediculi, or lice*, which infest the body. For this purpose 80 grains of the seeds, divested of shell, should be beaten up into a paste in a mortar, and then thoroughly incorporated with an ounce of lard, kokum butter, or ghee. In applying this ointment, care should be taken to avoid all abraded or ulcerated surfaces, on account of the danger of absorption of the poisonous principle of the seeds.

108. Sulphate of Copper. Blue Stone.

Nílá-tútá (*Hind. Punj.*), Mór-tuttá, Mhor-tuttah (*Duk.*), Tutiyá (*Beng.*), Nila-toth (*Kash.*), Mayil-tuttam, Turichu, Tuttam-turichi (*Tam.*), Mayilu-tuttam (*Tel.*), Turisha, Mayil-tutta (*Mal.*), Mail-tutyá (*Can.*), Mórtúta (*Guz.*), Palmánikam (*Cing.*), Douthá (*Burm.*), Toorsi (*Malay*).

109. Sulphate of Copper, of fair quality, is procurable in most bazaars; it should be in crystalline masses, of various sizes, of a dark-blue colour, without any light-green or whitish powder adherent on the surface; if these exist they should be thoroughly removed previous to the salt being employed medicinally. Or it may be further purified by dissolving in boiling water, filtering, and setting the solution aside to crystallize. In doses of from a quarter grain

to two grains it acts as an astringent and tonic; in larger doses (5 to 10 grains) it is a powerful emetic.

110. *In Chronic Diarrhœa and Dysentery* the following pills are often productive of great benefit. Take finely powdered Sulphate of Copper and Opium, of each 6 grains; thoroughly mix them with a small portion of honey, and divide into twelve pills, of which one should be taken thrice daily. These pills have been found very useful in controlling *Diarrhœa in the advanced stages of Consumption (Phthisis). In the Chronic Diarrhœa and Dysentery of Children,* a better form is 2 grains of the Sulphate dissolved in 12 drachms of Omum water; of this the dose is a tea spoonful thrice daily. In all these cases, should benefit not be manifest in a few days, the remedy should be discontinued.

111. *In Diphtheria* the Sulphate of Copper has been highly spoken of. Of a solution of 5 grains in one ounce of water, a tea spoonful may be given to young children, and repeated every half hour till it produces vomiting. The same treatment has also been advised in cases of *Croup.* After the occurrence of free vomiting, its use should be discontinued.

112. *In Ulcerations of the Mouth,* whether occurring in children or adults, 3 to 5 grains of finely powdered Sulphate, incorporated with half an ounce of honey, are a very useful application. It may be easily applied to the ulcers by the finger.

113. *In the Ophthalmia of Children attended with copious discharge,* a solution of one grain in one ounce of water, applied several times in the day, will often be found serviceable. In obstinate cases the strength

may be doubled, but it should never be so strong as to cause pain.

114. *Obstinate Indolent Ulcers* will often yield, when other measures have failed, to the persevering application of solutions of the Sulphate, of graduated strengths, from 2 grains to 10 grains in the ounce of water. At the commencement the weakest solution is applied morning and evening, water dressing (394) being applied in the intervals. When the first solution ceases to occasion a feeling of heat in the ulcerated surface, the strength should be gradually increased by single grains till the 10-grain solution is borne, by which time the ulcer is generally almost healed. When the edges of the ulcer are hard and unyielding, they may be touched every second or third day with the Sulphate in substance; and it may also be thus used to check *Exuberant Granulations.*

115. *In Ring worm* and *Scald head* the following ointment has been found useful: Sulphate of Copper in powder, 20 grains; powdered Galls, 1 drachm; Lard or Ceromel, 1 ounce. Mix them thoroughly, and rub well into the diseased spot. *In Prickly Heat,* a lotion of the Sulphate of Copper (10 grains to one ounce of water, or Rose water) often affords more relief than any other application.

116. *Excessive Bleeding from Leech bites* may often be speedily arrested by the application of a little powdered Sulphate of Copper. *In Bleeding from the Nose,* a solution of 4 grains of the Sulphate in one ounce of water introduced into the nostril, is sometimes effectual when Alum fails.

117. *In poisoning by Opium, Datura, Nux Vomica, Cocculus Indicus, Bish* (*Aconite*), *Arsenic, &c.*, where the poison has been swallowed, an emetic should at once be given to evacuate the contents of the stomach. For this purpose, Sulphate of Copper may be advantageously employed—5 grains in a pint of tepid water, taken at a draught. If this does not operate in half an hour it may be repeated; and a third dose, even, may be given if necessary, but this quantity should not be exceeded; as, unless it is vomited up, it remains in the stomach, and in large quantities is itself capable of acting as a poison. Its operation should be promoted by copious draughts of warm water. Its use, as an emetic, should be limited to cases of poisoning when it is of the greatest importance to empty the stomach as rapidly as possible. In other cases it is not a safe or manageable emetic. White of egg is the best remedy, if it causes any unpleasant effects.

118. **Croton Seeds.** The seeds of Croton Tiglium, *Linn.*

Jépál, Jamál-gótá (*Hind.*), Jamál-guttah (*Duk.*), Jépál, Jamál-gotá (*Beng. Punj.*), Nérválam-kottai (*Tam.*), Népála-vittulu (*Tel.*), Nirválam (*Mal.*), Jápálada-bíjá (*Can.*), Népálácha-bi (*Mah.*), Jamlá-gota (*Guz.*), Jápála, Jaipála (*Cing.*), Kanakho-si, Sa-díva, Ta-díva (*Burm.*), Buah doomkian (*Malay*).

119. The Croton seeds, met with in Indian bazaars, are often spoilt by long keeping, &c.; they should, when practicable, be collected fresh when required for

use. They are about the size of a grain of coffee, oval, rounded, of an imperfectly quadrangular form, with a thin brittle light-coloured shell, containing a yellowish albuminous kernel, enclosing a large leafy embryo; inodorous; taste at first mild, subsequently acrid and pungent. In their natural state they are violently purgative, and even in small quantity poisonous.

120. The following Croton pill is said to be an effectual purgative: Take any quantity of the seeds, deprived of their outer shell, boil them three times in milk, and after boiling, carefully remove the outer skin and the little leaf-like body (embryo), which will be found between the two halves of the kernel; if the latter be allowed to remain, it will cause violent griping and vomiting. To 30 grains of the seeds thus prepared add 60 grains of finely-powdered Catechu, and with the aid of a little honey or gum beat them into an even mass. Mix the ingredients thoroughly, and divide into pills, each weighing two grains. One of these is a sufficient dose for an adult, and should be given only when a strong purgative is required, as in *Apoplexy*, *Convulsions*, *Insanity*, *Ardent Fevers*, &c. Should it cause much griping, vomiting, or too violent purging, a good large draught of lime juice is the best remedy; and it may be safely repeated in half an hour if the vomiting, &c., continue.

121. The oil expressed from these seeds, CROTON OIL, is a powerful purgative, in doses of one drop, or even less, made into a pill, with bread-crumb. It is applicable for all the cases mentioned in the last section; and where one drop does not operate, the

dose may be increased to two, or even three drops. In *Apoplexy*, *Fits*, &c., where the patient is unable to swallow, it is sufficient to place the oil at the base of the tongue. Its use, as a general rule, should be confined to adults.

122. A useful stimulant liniment is made by mixing half an ounce of Croton Oil with three and a half ounces of Sesamum, Cocoa-nut, or other bland oil. It causes a vesicular eruption, and proves serviceable in *Chronic Rheumatism*, *Paralysis*, *Diseases of the Joints*, *Phthisis*, and *Chronic Bronchitis*.

123. **Cubebs.** The dried unripe fruit of Cubeba officinalis, *Miquel.*

Kabáb-chíní (*Hind.*, *Duk.*, *Punj.*), Liút-marz (*Kash.*), Vál-milagu (*Tam.*), Tóka-miriyálu, Chalava-miriyálu (*Tel.*), Vál-mulaka (*Mal.*), Bála-menasu (*Can.*), Kabábachini, Himsí-míre (*Mah.*), Kabáb-chíní, Tadamirí (*Guz.*), Vál-molagu, Vát-molavú (*Cing.*), Lada-bereker (*Malay*).

124. Cubebs of very fair quality is often obtainable in the bazaars.* It is usually about the size of black

* In Southern India and elsewhere, *Sital-Chíní* is the name in use for Cubebs, and *Kabáb-chíní* for Allspice (fruit of Eugenia Pimenta) whereas in Calcutta the reverse holds good, the former (*Sital-Chíní*) is applied to Allspice, and the latter (*Kabáb-chíní*) to Cubebs. In the Madras bazaars, the name Kabáb-chíní is also often applied to the buds of *Mesua ferrea:* this is incorrect, the proper name of the latter being *Nágésar* (Moodeen Sheriff). According to Dr. Aitchison the fruit of Xanthoxylon hastile, *Wall*, is often sold as Cubebs (Kabab-chíní) in the Punjab bazaars.

pepper, globular, wrinkled, blackish, supported on a short stalk, has an acrid camphoraceous taste, and a peculiar aromatic odour. Within the shell is a hard, spherical, whitish, oily kernel.

125. The chief use of Cubebs is as a remedy in *Gonorrhœa*, but it is only admissible in the more advanced stages, when the acute symptoms have subsided; in the earlier stages it may do harm. The following is a good form: Take of powdered Cubebs, two ounces; powdered Alum, half an ounce. Mix thoroughly, and divide into nine equal parts, one to be taken thrice daily in water. These powders may also be used with benefit in *Gleet, Leucorrhœa, and other Vaginal Discharges in Women.*

126. *The Coughs of Old Age*, attended with much expectoration, are sometimes greatly benefited by Cubebs in doses of eight or ten grains thrice daily.

127. **Datura.** The dried leaves and stems of Datura alba, *Linn.*, and Datura fastuosa, *Linn.*

Dhatúrá (*Hind., Duk., Beng., Punj., Guz.*), Umattai (*Tam.*), Dáthir (*Kash.*), Ummetta, Duttúramu (*Tel.*), Ummatta (*Mal.*), Ummatte (*Can.*), Attana (*Cing.*), Padáyin (*Burm.*), Kachubung (*Malay*). These are the native generic names of the Datura plant, the different species being distinguished by affixes denoting the colour of the flowers, white, purple, &c.

128. The white and purple varieties of Datura are common on waste places throughout India; they

possess the same medicinal properties, and although the purple variety is generally regarded as the more powerful, there is no evidence of its being so. Although a valuable medicine, much caution is necessary in its employment; as in over-doses it acts as a powerful narcotic poison. A very useful preparation is a Tincture made by macerating two and a half ounces of bruised Datura seeds in one pint of Proof Spirit (356) for seven days in a closed vessel, occasionally shaking; it should then be pressed, and filtered, and measured, and sufficient Proof Spirit added to make one pint. This Tincture generally produces all the sedative and narcotic effects which could be expected from Opium, besides effecting a great saving; Opium being very expensive, whilst this tincture can be prepared at a comparatively small cost. The dose requires to be regulated in each individual case; it is better, therefore, to commence with small doses of ten or twelve drops in a little water, and increase them to twenty or thirty drops, according to circumstances. As a general rule, twenty drops will be found to be equal in effect to one grain of Opium. One of the effects of Datura is to produce dilatation of the pupil; the eye should therefore be occasionally examined whilst this remedy is being administered, and should the pupil be found very large and dilated, it may be regarded as a sign that the medicine has been carried as far as it can be with safety, whether it has produced its other intended effects or not.

128β. In Datura we have an excellent, if not perfect, indigenous substitute for Belladonna in the treatment of *Cataract and other Diseases of the Eye.* Its mydriatic (pupil-dilating) powers have been examined by Sub-Assist. Surgeon Tarra Prosonno Roy (*Indian Med. Gaz.* Sept. 1870). He first applied a portion of a watery extract of the leaves of D. alba around the eyes; the pupils became widely dilated, and continued so for two days. He next tried an alcoholic extract of the seeds of the same species prepared by macerating half an ounce of the seeds in four ounces of country spirit, evaporating the tincture to dryness on a water bath, and dissolving the residue in one ounce of water. Experiments made with this solution prove beyond a doubt its power of causing dilatation of the pupil when locally applied; the strength of this watery solution being, at a rough estimate, about equal in power to a four grain (to the ounce) solution of Atropine.

129. *In Asthma,* the dried leaves and stem cut small and smoked, like tobacco, in a pipe, afford in many cases great relief. In some the benefit is immediate and striking, in others it has little effect, and in a few it acts injuriously; its value in any case can only be ascertained by personal experiment, but it is worth a trial in all cases. When the leaves fail, the dried seeds, which are thought to be more powerful, may be tried. The earlier in the attack it is employed the greater are the chances of success; it has little effect when the attack has lasted for some hours. For a person subject to asthma, a good plan is to adopt the habit of smoking a pipe of it the last thing at night, whether an attack is threatening or not; at any rate,

he should keep a pipe of it already filled, with the means of lighting it, by his bedside, so that, immediately on an attack commencing, he may use it. From ten to twenty grains of the dried plant is sufficient to commence with; it may subsequently be increased to thirty grains, but in all cases it should be immediately discontinued if it produces giddiness, a feeling of sickness, or any other unpleasant symptom. Serious, and even fatal, consequences have followed its incautious use, hence too much care cannot be exercised in its employment. In *Chronic Coughs*, where the cough comes on in violent paroxysms, and is hard and dry, with scanty expectoration, smoking Datura (*ante*) proves beneficial.

130. *For Rheumatic Swellings of the Joints, Lumbago, Painful Tumours, Nodes*, &c., Datura, locally applied, often proves most serviceable in relieving pain. There are four modes, in either of which it may be advantageously employed: 1. POULTICE, made by bruising the fresh leaves into a pulp, and mixing them, with the aid of a little water, with an equal weight of rice flour, to the consistence of a poultice. 2. EPITHEM; which consists of steeping a few entire leaves in arrack or other spirit, and placing them, whilst wet, over the seat of pain, and securing them in that position by a bandage. 3. FOMENTATION; made by infusing the leaves in boiling water, in the proportion of one ounce to each pint of fluid, and applying as directed in paragraph 393. 4. LINIMENT; prepared by macerating, for seven days, one ounce of the bruised seeds in a pint of Sesamum or other bland oil, and straining.

In addition to the above-named affections, these preparations, applied to the loins, are useful in relieving *the Pain attendant on painful or difficult Menstruation*, and in some *painful affections of the Uterus;* in the latter, they may more advantageously be placed over the lower part of the abdomen. They also prove beneficial in relieving *Neuralgic pains, especially of the Face;* for this the liniment is best adapted, well rubbed in over the seat of pain, and along the space immediately in front of the ear, or rather, in the narrow space between the ears and the jaw.

131. *In Tetanus or Lock-jaw, consequent on a wound,* Datura is worthy of a trial in the absence of more effective agents.* Poultices of the leaves, renewed three or four times a-day, should be kept constantly to the wound, which should be further cleansed if covered with thick discharge or slough, by the process of irrigation of tepid water (395). The Tincture of Datura, in doses of 20 to 30 drops in water, may also be given internally three or four times daily. The dose must be regulated by the effect produced, but it may be continued, unless the spasms previously yield, till it produces full dilatation of the pupil with some degree of giddiness, drowsiness, or confusion of ideas, beyond which it is not safe to carry the medicine. If

* The treatment detailed in this paragraph is advocated from the success which has in some cases of Tetanus attended the use of Belladonna — a drug to which Datura bears a very close resemblance in its effects on the system: employed as above directed, it may be used with perfect safety, provided that the case is carefully watched, and the medicine diminished or discontinued on the full development of its physiological effects.

the spasms abate, *i.e.*, if they recur at more distant intervals, and are less severe and prolonged when they do occur, the medicine, in smaller doses at longer intervals, may be continued till the spasms cease altogether; but if, under the use of the remedy, after it has produced its specific effects on the system, the spasms show no sign of abatement, no good, but perhaps harm, will result from continuing it. In addition to the above means, Datura liniment (130) should be well rubbed in along the spine several times daily. The patient should be confined to a darkened room and protected from cold draughts of air; the bowels should be opened, if necessary by turpentine enemas (364). The strength should be supported by strong beef-tea, or mutton-broth (413), by eggs beaten up with milk, and by brandy-mixture (420), or other stimulants; if these cannot be swallowed they should be given in enemas, for which purpose not more than four ounces should be used at a time; larger quantities will not be retained.

132. *In cases of Guinea Worm*, a Datura poultice (130) is said to be the most useful in relieving the pain, and hastening the expulsion of the worm.

133. **Dill Seeds.** The fruit of Anethum Sowa, *Roxb.*

Sóyah, Suvà (*Hind.*, *Punj.*), Sóyí (*Duk.*), Sóí-biól (*Kash.*), Shulphà, Shonvá, Shóvá (*Beng.*), Shatta-kuppi-virai (*Tam.*), Shata-kuppi-víttulu (*Tel.*), Shata-kuftá (*Mal.*), Sab-basagi (*Can.*), Suvá-nu-bi (*Guz.*), Sada-kuppa, Sata-kuppi (*Cing.*), Samin (*Burm.*), Shatha-kupay, Adas pudus (*Malay*).

134. The Indian Dill Seed possesses no specific characters to distinguish it from the European article, for which it may be substituted. The Distilled Water, when procurable, is the best form, but in its absence an infusion of the bruised seeds, 3 drachms to half a pint of hot water, may be used; of this, when strained and cold, the dose for an infant is a dessert-spoonful or more, sweetened with a little sugar. It proves very effectual in relieving *Abdominal Pain, Flatulence, and Colic in Children.* Its efficacy is often much increased by the addition of a teaspoonful of lime water.

135. Fish-liver Oil.

Mach-chí-ká-tél (*Hind., Duk.*), Machár-tail (*Beng.*), Mín-yenney (*Tam.*), Chépa-núne (*Tel.*), Mínnai, Malsyam-nai (*Mal.*), Míniná-yanne (*Can.*), Mo-solícha-téla (*Mah.*), Mín-tel, Mal-tel (*Cing.*), Miniak bati-yu putch (*Malay*).

136. Oil from the livers of the White Shark (Squalus Carcharias, *Linn.*), the Seir (Cybium Commersonii, *Cuv. et Val.*), and other fish, is now extensively prepared in various sea-coast towns of India. When properly made it is of a fine amber colour; the smell and taste are similar to Cod-liver Oil, but more strongly marked and more disagreeable. The great objection to its use is its nauseous taste, but this might probably, in a great measure, be obviated by extracting it by the process of boiling the *fresh* livers in water, instead of allowing them to undergo a degree

of putrefaction before the process of extraction is commenced, as is the usual practice. As a medicinal agent it appears to be quite equal to Cod-liver Oil, for which it forms an excellent substitute; but where the stomach is very irritable, and the aversion to it unconquerable, it may be advisable to have recourse to the European imported article.*

137. *Remarks on its Use.* *a.* The best time for administering the oil is immediately after, or to those who prefer it during, a solid meal. Taken on an empty stomach it is almost sure to nauseate. Patients who can take it at no other time will sometimes retain a dose if given the last thing before going to bed.

b. For disguising the nauseous taste and preventing subsequent eructations, a good plan is to take a few grains of common salt, both immediately before and after a dose. As a vehicle, a little orange-wine,

* 'Turtle Oil,' prepared from 'turtles' (tortoises?) which abound in the Straits of Manaar, between India and Ceylon, has been proposed by native surgeon, Y. Anthony Pillay (*Madras Jour. of Med. Sci.*, March 1870) as a substitute for Cod-liver Oil, over which it has the advantage of being four times cheaper. After two years' experience of it in dispensary practice he reported highly of its efficacy in that large class of scrofulous and anæmic cases in which fish-oil is indicated. Specimens of this oil sent to the Madras Medical Stores were pronounced unfit for medicinal use; but the principal storekeeper (Dr. F. Day) adds, 'If this turtle oil were prepared from the animal after it had been well cleansed from all blood, and the straining properly carried out, an oil would probably be produced but little inferior to the present fish-oil.' It seems well worthy of notice in the southern portion of the Peninsula, where it is procurable at very small cost.

or solution of quinine, or lime juice, or hot strong coffee without milk, has been advocated by various writers. A little Omum water (317) is perhaps the best vehicle of all.

c. The bulk of the whole dose of the oil and vehicle together should be so small that it may be swallowed at a single draught; therefore the vehicle should not exceed a table spoonful, with, at first, a tea spoonful of the oil, to be gradually increased to a table spoonful. The spoon and glass used for taking it should be kept scrupulously clean, as any oil left adhering to them soon turns rancid. In taking this (as well as all other nauseous drugs) it is advisable to prevent, as far as possible, the tongue from coming in contact with it; to effect this the tongue should be projected on the surface of the glass or spoon, and the fluid thrown down as far back in the throat as can conveniently be done.

d. The dose, as a general rule, at the commencement is a tea spoonful three times daily, gradually increased as the stomach is able to bear it. It is rarely requisite to exceed a table spoonful twice or thrice daily; large quantities either derange the stomach and liver, or pass off unabsorbed by the bowels.

e. The diet during the course of the oil should be plain and nutritious, consisting of bread, fresh meat roast or boiled, poultry, game, &c., with a fair proportion of vegetables, and fruit, and a moderate quantity of liquids. All rich articles of food, as pastry, fat meat, cream, &c., should be avoided. Wine is preferable to beer, the latter often disagreeing. Should a bilious attack come on, the oil should be discontinued, the diet lightened, and an occasional aperient administered. In a few days, when the attack has passed off, the oil may be resumed, beginning with the small doses as at the first. In all cases during the use of the oil, the bowels should be kept regular, if necessary, by mild aperients.

f. During its use the patient should be as much as possible in the open air, and take gentle exercise.

138. It is *in Pulmonary Consumption* that the value of Fish-liver Oil is most manifest, but there are a large number of cases of a scrofulous character in which it proves almost equally valuable. *In Scrofulous Abscesses, Suppurating Glands, Ulcerations, Discharges, whether from the nose or ears, and Skin Diseases,* especially when the patient is weak and emaciated, the oil is indicated and proves most beneficial. It proves equally useful in *Scrofulous Affections of the Joints and Bones,* especially in *Rickets;* and in *Scrofulous Ophthalmia.*

139. *In the Mesenteric Affections of Children* the best results often follow its use; the little patient rapidly gains strength and flesh, the tumefied belly becomes reduced, the stools lose their clayey colour and become bilious and healthy. It should not only be given internally, but should be used as a liniment to the abdomen. *The Obstinate Constipation of Children* sometimes yields to the use of the oil, and its return is prevented while the remedy is continued. *In Stricture of the Rectum,* as an adjunct to dilatation cod-liver oil is an excellent remedy: it nourishes the patient, and

softens the motions, rendering aperients unnecessary. (*Mr. Curling.*) It is also well worthy of a trial in cases of *Chronic Hydrocephalus, or Water on the Brain,* occurring in children of a scrofulous habit.

140. *In the advanced stages of Hooping Cough, and in other Spasmodic Coughs, which often remain after an attack of Bronchitis,* especially when occurring in weakly children, marked benefit follows its use.

141. *Chorea (St. Vitus's Dance) and Epilepsy* sometimes are benefited by it when more active remedies have failed. The same remark applies to some forms of *Neuralgia,* especially *Tic Douloureux;* but the cases in which it will prove serviceable can only be ascertained by trials with the remedy.

142. *In Chronic Rheumatism* attended with much debility and emaciation, it often proves useful; in fact, in all cases of *Atrophy (wasting or emaciation), whether connected with Rheumatism, Scrofula or defective digestion or resulting from long-continued confinement in close rooms, as in jails,* &c., a course of the oil offers the best prospects of success. In some form of *Paralysis* it is occasionally very beneficial. *In Leprosy* it is a remedy well worthy of careful trial; not so much as a curative agent as a means of relieving many of the distressing symptoms.

143. In all the above cases the remedy should be persevered in for weeks or even longer; and the rules given above for its administration must be carefully attended to. Its operation is most beneficial in the cold season.

144. **Galls.**

Mái-phal, Mázú-phal (*Hind.*), Mái-phal, Májú-phal (*Duk.*), Máju-phal (*Beng.*, *Punj.*, *Kash.*), Máshik-káy (*Tam.*), Máshi-káya (*Tel.*), Máshik-káya (*Mal.*), Máchi-káyi (*Can.*), Mái-phala, Máshi-ká (*Mah.*), Máyi-phal (*Guz.*), Mása-ka (*Cing.*), Pinza-káni-si, Pinz-gáni-di (*Burm.*), Manjakani (*Malay*).

145. Many varieties of Galls are met with in the bazaars; the best for medical use are globular, about the size of a nutmeg, of a yellowish-white colour and very astringent taste, with a small hole on one side of the surface. In the absence of this kind the other varieties of Galls may be employed, as they all partake, more or less, of the same astringent qualities. The dose for an adult is from 10 to 20 grains in powder or infusion; but a better form is Decoction, prepared by boiling for ten minutes in an earthenware vessel 1½ ounces of bruised Galls in a pint of Water; of this, when cold and strained, the dose is from 1 to 2 ounces thrice daily, or oftener. This decoction forms also a useful astringent wash, gargle, &c.

146. *In Chronic Diarrhœa, especially in Natives,* powdered Galls in 15 grain doses thrice daily often prove useful, and in obstinate cases its efficacy is increased by the addition of half a grain of Opium with each dose. A little powdered Cinnamon may be advantageously added, and the whole given in honey. *In the advanced stages of Dysentery* the decoction (*ante*) seems to answer better, and it may be given in doses of 1½ to 2 ounces thrice daily, with the addition of

F

Opium, as above, and a carminative. This treatment is adapted only for adults.

147. *In Prolapsus (Descent) of the Rectum*, the daily use of an enema of decoction of Galls proves useful by constringing the parts; and this may further be effected, especially in the case of children, by keeping a pad saturated with the decoction over the external parts after the protruded bowel has been returned. The same treatment is applicable (the decoction being used as a vaginal injection) in cases of *Prolapsus of the Uterus* (*Descent of the Womb*).

148. *In Piles unattended by increased heat or inflammation*, a very useful application is an ointment composed of 1½ drachms of powdered Galls, and 1 ounce of Ghee. The ingredients should be thoroughly mixed. If there should be much pain half a drachm of Opium may be added to it. It should be applied twice daily. Enemas of the decotion (*ante*) may also be used with advantage.

149. *In Gleet and long standiug Gonorrhœa*, 20 grains of powdered Galls, twice or thrice daily, have sometimes a good effect in checking the discharge. *In Leucorrhœa, and other Vaginal Discharges*, the same treatment is applicable, and at the same time injections of the decoction may be employed.

150. *In Relaxed sore Throat and Enlargement of the Tonsils* a very useful gargle is composed of 40 grains of Alum, six ounces of Decoction of Galls (145), and one ounce of Honey.

151. *In the Intermittent Fevers of Natives*, powdered Galls, in doses of 20 to 30 grains, three or four times

a day, have been found serviceable in some cases; or smaller doses (10 to 12 grains) may be given in $1\frac{1}{2}$ ounces of Infusion of Chiretta (98) repeated every hour, for four or five times in succession, immediately before the period at which the fever usually returns. An aperient should, in all cases, be taken before commencing this treatment, which is only suited for adults.

152. *In Poisoning by Nux Vomica, Cocculus Indicus, Datura, Opium, and Bish* (*Aconite Root*), after the stomach has been freely emptied by emetics (which is the first thing to be done), the Decoction of Galls, in doses of 3 or 4 ounces, should be given every ten minutes or quarter of an hour, for four or five times in succession. It is thought to act as an antidote; in some cases it certainly seems to act very beneficially.

153. **Ginger.** The dried root of Zingiber officinalis, *Roscoe.*

Sónth, Sindhi (*Hind.*), Sónth (*Duk.*, *Beng.*, *Punj.*), Shó-ont (*Kash.*), Shukku (*Tam.*), Sonti (*Tel.*), Chukka (*Mal.*), Vanasunthi (*Can.*), Súnt (*Guz.*), Ingúrú, Velichaingúrú (*Cing.*), Ginsi-khiáv (*Burm.*), Hulya-kring (*Malay*).

154. Dried Ginger is preferable to fresh or green Ginger for medicinal use, but if not procurable the latter may be employed. It is best given in the form of Infusion, made by macerating 1 ounce of bruised Ginger in a pint of boiling water in a covered vessel for an hour and straining. The dose is from 1 to 2

ounces. A very useful domestic remedy is made by steeping 3 ounces of Ginger in a pint of Brandy for ten days. Of this a tea spoonful or more may, with great advantage, be added to aperient, antacid and other medicines.

155. *In Colic, Flatulence, Vomiting, Spasms and other painful Affections of the Bowels unattended by fever*, the above Infusion, especially if taken warm, in doses of 2 ounces every half-hour or hour, often affords great relief. The addition of 20 or 30 grains of Carbonate of Soda, if at hand, greatly increases its efficacy. For children a table spoonful of the infusion is sufficient.

156. *In Chronic Rheumatism* Infusion of Ginger (2 drachms to 6 ounces of boiling water and strained), taken warm the last thing before going to bed, the body being covered with blankets so as to produce copious perspiration, is often attended with the best effects. The same treatment has also been found very beneficial in *Colds or Catarrhal attacks*, and during *the cold stage of Intermittent Fever.*

157. *In Headache* a Ginger plaister, made by bruising Ginger with a little water to the consistence of a poultice, applied to the forehead, affords in many instances much relief. *Toothache and Faceache* are sometimes relieved by the same application to the face.

158. *Relaxed Sore Throat, Hoarseness*, and *Loss of Voice*, are sometimes benefited by chewing a piece of Ginger so as to produce a copious flow of saliva.

159. **Gurjun Balsam, or Wood Oil.** The balsamic exudation of Dipterocarpus lævis, *Ham.*

Garjan-ká-tél (*Hind.*), Gorjon-tail (*Beng.*), Hora-tel (*Cing.*), Kanyen-si (*Burm.*).

160. Gurjun Balsam, or Wood Oil, is a transparent liquid of the consistence of olive oil, lighter than water, of a dark-brown sherry colour, with an odour and taste resembling Copaiba, but less powerful. It has been used as a substitute for this latter drug in the treatment of *Gonorrhœa*, and trials with it in the hands of Europeans have shown that it is a remedy of no mean value in this affection. It is only advisable in the advanced stages, or when the disease has degenerated into *Gleet.* In the latter affection it is stated to prove most useful. It is also well worthy of a trial in *Leucorrhœa and other Vaginal Discharges.* The dose is about a tea spoonful twice or thrice daily, given floating on Omum or other aromatic water, or made into an emulsion with lime water. It is apt occasionally to produce an eruption on the skin similar to that which, in some instances, follows the use of Copaiba.

161. *In Leprosy* the use of Gurjum Balsam was introduced in 1873 by Surgeon-Major J. Dougall, and the reported success of the remedy gave rise to sanguine anticipations that a specific for this disease had at last been discovered. Although subsequent experience proved this hope to be fallacious, yet the lessons imparted by Dr. Dougall's treatment are far from unimportant. His treatment consisted in the internal

and external use of the Balsam : for the former purpose it was given in two drachm doses, with lime-water, twice daily : for the latter, in the form of ointment composed of 1 part of the Balsam and 3 of lime-water, which was directed to *be thoroughly and perseveringly rubbed in over the whole body for two hours a day by the patient himself, as far as practicable.* This was insisted upon not only for the sake of the action of the ointment on the skin, but because it was considered that any gentle employment conjoined with exercise was likely to prove beneficial both physically and mentally. Under this treatment (no change having been made in the diet) Dr. Dougall obtained signal and manifest improvement in numerous cases; but this was unhappily found to be of only a temporary character, the discontinuance of the remedy being in all cases followed by a relapse. Still further to test this treatment, Dr. A. H. Hilson (*Indian Ann. of Med. Sci.*, Jan. 1877) instituted two sets of trials on leprous subjects (12 of each group), treated respectively by Gurjun Balsam, used externally and internally on Dr. Dougall's system, and by the ordinary Til (Sesamum) or Sweet Oil of the bazaars, used externally only. The results which he arrived at are as follows : 1. That the application of Gurjun oil removes the local manifestations of leprosy to a great extent. 2. That it has no specific influence over the constitutional taint or leprous cachexia. 3. That ordinary Sweet Oil is equally efficacious as far as the local effect is concerned, and therefore it is not improbable that the benefit which patients experience from the application of Gurjun oil is due to the friction producing absorption of the deposits which are effused into the skin and cellular tissue during the course of the disease. Dr. Dougall may have failed in finding in Gurjun oil a specific in leprosy, but he has rendered important service in leading us to a knowledge of the vast benefits to be derived from diligent oleaginous frictions in its treatment; and, as he himself justly remarks, 'even temporary improvement is worth striving after in such a disease.'

161*a*. **Hemidesmus Root,** or **Country Sarsaparilla.** The root of Hemidesmus Indicus, *R. Brown.*

Híndí-sál-sá, Jangli-chanbéllí (*Hind.*), Nanníré-jar (*Duk.*), Ananto-múl (*Beng.*), Nannárí-vér (*Tam.*), Sugandhi-pála, Pála-chukkam-déru (*Tel.*), Nannári-kizhanna, Naru-níntí (*Mal.*), Sugandha-pálada-béru (*Can.*), Irimusu (*Cing.*).

162. The specimens of Hemidesmus Root, procurable in most parts of India, which are best adapted for medical use are medium sized, about the size of a quill, having a full, peculiar aromatic odour, and a feebly bitter and agreeable taste. The freshly collected root is preferable to that bought in the bazaars, as that is often inodorous, tasteless, and almost worthless. The virtues of the drug reside mainly in the root-bark, hence if the larger roots are employed you get an undue proportion of the inner woody portion, which is comparatively inert.

163. Hemidesmus proves most useful in *Constitu-*

tional Debility, from whatever cause arising; also in *Chronic Rheumatism, Constitutional Syphilis, Skin Diseases and Ulcerations, especially those of Syphilitic origin, Indigestion*, and *Loss of Appetite.* It is best given in the form of Infusion, prepared by infusing one ounce of the bruised roots in half a pint of boiling water in a covered vessel for an hour, and straining. Of this the dose is from 2 to 3 ounces thrice daily. Its efficacy is much increased by being taken while the Infusion is still warm; the addition of milk and sugar renders it so like ordinary tea that children will take it readily; and this is fortunate, as it is a peculiarly useful tonic for the pale, weakly offspring of Europeans in India; for such it may be substituted for tea at breakfast and supper. Some children prefer it to ordinary tea.

164. **Honey.**

Shahad, Madh (*Hind.*), Shahad (*Duk.*), Modhu (*Beng.*), Tén (*Tam.*), Téne (*Tel.*), Tén (*Mal.*), Jénu (*Can.*), Mada (*Mah.*), Madh (*Guz.*), Páni (*Cing.*), Piyá-ye (*Burm.*), Ayer madu (*Malay*), Saht, Shahd (*Punj.*), Mhách (*Kash.*).

165. Honey of fair quality is obtainable in most parts of India. Though not possessed of any marked medicinal properties, it is always advisable to keep some in store, as it forms an agreeable sweetening ingredient for mixtures, is a good vehicle in which to administer powders for children, and is one of the best substances in making pills, &c. Should it be dirty

and impure, it should be 'clarified' by melting in a water bath and straining through cloth.

166. A mixture of Honey and Distilled Vinegar or Lime juice, in equal parts, melted together by gentle heat, is an excellent adjunct to cough mixtures; and in the *Coughs of Childhood* this combination, diluted with an equal quantity of water, and with or without a few drops of Paregoric, forms a useful and pleasant mixture, which children will readily take when they will not swallow other more nauseous medicines.

167. An excellent stimulant application, termed CEROMEL, for *Indolent and other Ulcerations*, is formed by melting together, with the aid of gentle heat, 1 ounce of Yellow Wax and 4 ounces of Clarified Honey, and straining. It is admirably adapted for use in hot climates, where animal fats, the basis of so many ointments, soon become rancid and unfit for medicinal use.

168. **Hydrocotyle Asiatica,** *Linn.*

Vallári (*Hind.*, *Duk.*), Thal-kúru (*Beng.*), Valláraí (*Tam.*), Mandúka-bramha-kúráku, Pinna-éaki-chettu, Bokkudu-chettu (*Tel.*), Kutakan, Kodogam (*Mal.*), Von-delagá *Can.*), Hingotu-kola (*Cing.*), Mink-hua-bin (*Burm.*), Dawoon-pungagah (*Malay*).

169. This small, low-growing plant, common in moist localities in many parts of India, has obtained considerable repute in European practice as a remedy for *Leprosy.* It is prepared as follóws: The leaves

having been carefully separated, as soon as possible after the plant is gathered, should be spread on a mat in the shade, and then freely exposed to the air, but not to the sun.* They lose about nine-tenths of weight by drying. When thoroughly dried they should be finely powdered and kept in well corked or stoppered bottles. Of this powder the dose is from 3 to 5 grains thrice daily. At the same time some of the powder may be sprinkled on the ulcers, or, which is better, poultices made of the fresh leaves bruised into a paste, may be applied. Under its use the patient, in the course of a few weeks, improves in all respects. After continuing its use for some time, this remedy causes great itching of the skin over the whole body; under these circumstances it should be discontinued for a week, aperients administered, and then the medicine recommenced. Though it may not effect a cure, it often does a great deal of good. It may also be tried in *Scrofula* and *Syphilis.*

170. *Chronic Ulcerations of Syphilitic and Scrofulous origin* often show a marked improvement under the internal and local use of this remedy, but it requires to be steadily persevered in.

171. Sulphate of Iron.

Hirá-kasis, Kashish (*Hind.*), Hírá-kashísh (*Duk.*), Hirákos, Hírá-kosis (*Beng.*), Sang-i-sabz (*Punj., Kash.*), Híra-kasis (*Guz.*), Anná-bédi, Anná-bhédi (*Tam., Tel., Mal., Can.*), Madu-kolpa (*Malay*).

* In preparing the powder for use, avoid using any heat, as this dissipates all its virtues.

172. Sulphate of iron, in a more or less pure state, is met with in most Indian bazaars; that only should be selected for medicinal use which occurs in the form of crystals or small crystalline masses of a pale green colour, wholly soluble in water. The dirty yellowish powder usually associated with it in bazaar specimens, as well as the flat whitish-yellow cakes sold under the same native names as the Sulphate, should be rejected. It is a valuable tonic and astringent in doses of from ¼ grain to 2 grains. In solution it forms a useful external application.

173. *Remarks on the use of this and other Preparations of Iron.*

a. Under its use the stools become black and offensive, but they resume their natural characters when the medicine is discontinued. The tongue also, if iron has been taken in solution, becomes black.

b. In order to judge fairly of its effects, it requires to be persevered in for weeks or longer.

c. No advantage is gained by giving it in large doses. The fact of the stools becoming deeply black is an indication that the dose may be diminished.

d. Purgatives increase its efficacy; a dose of castor oil, or other aperient, every week or ten days, is advisable during a course of Iron.

e. Acids and acidulous fruits should be avoided during its use.

f. Children may take it not only with safety, but with advantage.

174. *In that form of Constitutional Debility termed Anæmia*, when the body is apparently bloodless, when, especially in natives, the inner surface of the eyelids, the tongue, and the palms of the hands, become very pale or white, the Sulphate proves very valuable. It is best given in solution as follows : Take of Sulphate of Iron, 4 grains, Omum water and Infusion of Chiretta, of each 6 ounces; of this the dose is a wine glassful thrice daily for adults, and from a tea spoonful to a table spoonful for children, according to age. Anæmic females, suffering from *Leucorrhœa* (*Whites*) and *Amenorrhœa* (*Suspension of menstrual discharge*), may advantageously take it combined with Aloes as advised in paragraph 18.

175. *In Intermittent Fever* the Sulphate often proves of great service, especially in obstinate or longstanding cases, where the patient has become weak and anæmic. It may be given as follows: Take of Sulphate of Iron, finely powdered, 24 grains; powdered Black Pepper, 30 grains; beat them into a mass with a little honey, and divide into twelve pills. Of these two should be taken twice or thrice daily, with a wineglassful of Infusion of Chiretta (98), or Gulancha (352). Whilst taking these pills, all acids and acidulous fruits should be avoided, and the bowels kept open. They are inadmissible when the stomach is very irritable, or when diarrhœa exists.

176. Long-continued or repeated attacks of *Intermittent Fever* are often accompanied by a swelling or hardness under the ribs of the left side; this constitutes the affection termed *Enlargement of the Spleen*

or *Ague Cake.* In these cases the treatment advised in the last paragraph may be resorted to with benefit, with the addition of a good active purgative once or twice a-week. Local pain may be relieved by Turpentine stupes or mustard poultices over the affected part.

177. *In Neuralgic or Rheumatic Faceache,* recurring periodically, especially when occurring in the weak and anæmic (174), Sulphate of Iron, in 2 or 3 grain doses thrice daily, produces excellent effects; it may be given in the form of pill, with a little Cinnamon powder and Honey, or in solution with Infusion of Chiretta (98), or Gulancha (352). *Chorea and other Nervous Affections* occurring in anæmic females are often greatly benefited by the Sulphate, conjoined with Aloes (18). *Paralysis and Rickets,* associated with anæmia, are likewise benefited by it.

178. *In Dropsy attended with Anæmia* (174) *and debility,* two grains of the Sulphate of Iron in a quart of water sweetened to taste, and taken in divided doses as an ordinary drink during the day, is a useful adjunct to other treatment.

179. *In Bleeding Piles, especially when the patient is much debilitated by the discharge,* daily enemas of the Sulphate, of the strength of 3 grains to 1 ounce of water, often prove of great service. The same treatment is well adapted for *Prolapsus (Descent) of the Rectum.*

180. *Obstinate Hooping Cough,* which resists Alum (28) and other remedies, sometimes yields to Sulphate of Iron in small and continued doses.

181. *In Chronic Diarrhœa* and *Dysentery of Childhood* in weak anæmic children the following mixture has been used with great advantage: Sulphate of Iron, 4 grains; Laudanum, 6 drops; Omum water, 10 drachms. Of this the dose is two tea spoonfuls every six hours for a child of one year of age, and so on in proportion.

182. **Jatamansi** or **Indian Spikenard.** The root of Nardostachys Jatamansi, *D. C.*

Jatámásí, Bál-chír (*Hind.*, *Punj.*), Jhatá-mánsí (*Duk.*), Jatámámsí (*Beng.*), Bhút-jatt, Kúkil-i-pót (*Kash.*), Jatámáshi (*Tam.*, *Tel.*), Jetá-mánchi (*Mal.*), Jetá-mávashí (*Can.*, *Mah.*), Jatamánsi, Jaramánsi (*Cing.*).

183. These roots, met with in most bazaars, occur in the form of short pieces of an underground stem, about the thickness of a goose quill, covered towards its tapering extremity, or almost entirely, with coarse, dark, hairlike fibres; odour, peculiar and fragrant; taste, aromatic and bitterish. In selecting specimens for medical use, care should be taken that they are fresh and of good quality; much of the drug sold in the bazaars being old, worm-eaten, and worthless.

184. Jatamansi is held in high repute by the natives as an antispasmodic, and trials made with it by Europeans tend to show that in this character it is a good substitute for the officinal Valerian; hence it is worthy of trial in *Hysterical Affections*, especially in

Palpitation of the Heart, Chorea, Flatulence, &c. It may be given in infusion (2 drachms of the bruised root to half-a-pint of boiling water, macerated for an hour and strained), in doses of a wine-glassful twice or thrice daily. A Tincture was ordered in the Bengal Pharmacopœia (5 ounces of bruised Jatamansi, Proof Spirit 2 pints), of which the dose is from 1 to 2 drachms. In all cases it may be advantageously combined with camphor, ammonia, and other remedies of the same class.

185. **Kala-dana.** The seeds of Pharbitis Nil, *Choisy.*

Kálá-dánah (*Hind.*), Kali-zirki-ká-bínj (*Duk.*), Kálá-dáná, Nil-kolomi (*Beng.*), Hub-úl-níl (*Punj., Kash.*), Kodi-kakkatán-virai, Jiriki-virai (*Tam.*), Jiriki-vittulu, Kolli-vittulu (*Tel.*).

186. Kala-dana seeds are black, angular, a quarter of an inch or more in length, weighing on an average about half a grain each, having the form of the segment of an orange; of a sweetish and subsequently rather acrid taste, and heavy smell.

187. The powdered seeds, in doses of from 30 to 50 grains, act as a safe and effectual purgative, forming an excellent substitute for Jalap, though not quite so active in its operation. When the ingredients are available, the following powder is preferable to the powdered seeds by themselves:—Powdered Kala-dana seeds, 7 drachms; Rock Salt; or Cream of Tartar, 7 drachms; powdered Ginger, 1 drachm. Rub

them well together in a mortar, and pass the powder through a fine sieve. Of this, the dose, as a purgative for an adult native, is from 60 to 90 grains. Somewhat less doses suffice for Europeans.

188. **Kamala** or **Kaméla.** The powder from the capsules of Mallotus Phillippiensis, *Müller.*

Kaméla, Kamúd (*Hind.*), Kaméla (*Beng.*), Kamélá-mávu, Kápila-podi (*Tam.*), Kápila-podi (*Tel.*), Kaméla (*Guz.*), Hampirilla-gedivella-buvá (*Cing.*), Rúlyá, Kamíla (*Punj.*), Kãim-bil (*Kash.*).

189. Kamala, much employed by the natives as a dye, is met with in most bazaars in the form of a beautiful purplish-red powder; it should be free from sand or earthy impurities. In medicine, it has attained considerable repute as a remedy for *Tœnia or Tape worm.* It has little or no effect on other forms of intestinal worms. The dose for an adult is from 2 to 3 drachms in honey, or a little aromatic water; no other medicine being necessary before or after. In the above doses it acts freely on the bowels, causing, in many instances, considerable nausea and griping, though not generally more than is caused by other remedies of the same class; the worm is generally expelled in a lifeless state in the third or fourth stool. Should the first trial not prove successful, it may be repeated after the interval of a week; but should this be a failure also, it will be useless to continue its use further; then other remedies may be tried.

190. **Kariyát** or **Creyat.** The dried stalks and root of Andrographis paniculata, *Nees.*

Charàyetah, Mahá-títá, Kiryat (*Hind.*), Charàyeta, Kalaf-náth (*Duk.*), Cherota, Mahá-tita (*Beng.*), Shirat-kúch-chi, Nila-vémbu (*Tam.*), Néla-vému (*Tel.*), Nila-véppa, Kiriyáttu (*Mal.*), Nela-bevinágidá (*Can.*), Chiráyita (*Mah.*), Kiryáta, Kiryáto (*Guz.*), Binko-hamba, Hín-binko-hamba (*Cing.*), Charita (*Malay*).

191. The stem, which is usually sold in the bazaars with the root attached, occurs in pieces of about a foot or more in length, quadrangular, of a lightish-brown colour, and persistent bitter taste. From the similarity between their native names and sensible qualities, this article is often confounded with Chiretta (96). Kariyát is a valuable bitter tonic, and may advantageously be employed in cases of *General Debility*, in *Convalescence after Fevers*, and in *the advanced stages of Dysentery.* It is best given as follows: Take of Kariyát, bruised, ½ ounce, Acorus, or Sweet Flag Root, and Dill Seeds bruised, of each 60 grains; Boiling Water, ½ pint; infuse in a covered vessel for an hour, and strain. Dose, from 1½ to 2 ounces twice or thrice daily.

192. The following preparation has been highly spoken of: Take of Kariyát, cut small, 6 ounces; Myrrh and Aloes, in coarse powder, of each 1 ounce; Brandy, 2 pints. Macerate for seven days in a closed vessel, occasionally shaking it, strain, press, filter, and add sufficient Brandy to make 2 pints. Of this the

dose is from one to four teaspoonfuls in a little water taken on an empty stomach. It acts as a gentle aperient, and is said to prove very useful in many forms of *Dyspepsia, especially when attended with torpidity of the bowels.*

193. *In the Bowel Complaints of Children* a decoction of the fresh leaves of the Kariyát plant has been well spoken of. It is prepared by boiling 2½ ounces of the fresh leaves in 1½ pints of water down to 6 ounces; of this the dose is one ounce every two or three hours. It may be used in conjunction with other remedies as required.

194. **Kokum Butter.** The concrete oil of the seeds of Garcinia purpurea, *Roxb.*

Kokam-ká-tél (*Hind.*).

195. This oil is obtained by first exposing the seeds to the action of the sun, when sufficiently dry bruising them, and then subjecting them to boiling; the oil collects on the surface, and on cooling, concretes into a solid cake. When purified it is rather brittle, of a pale yellowish colour, bland and mild to the taste, melting in the mouth, and leaving an impression of cold on the tongue. It melts at 98° F. From its bland, unirritating properties, as well as from its consistence, it seems admirably adapted for replacing animal fats in the preparation of ointments, &c. Were it largely produced, which it unfortunately is not, it might be extensively utilised in tropical pharmacy.

196. **Lawsonia alba,** *Linn.*, or **Henna Shrub.**

Mhíndí (*Hind.*), Mhéndí or Méndhí (*Duk.*, *Punj.*), Méhedi (*Beng.*), Móhnz (*Kash.*), Marutónri, Aivanam (*Tam.*), Góranta (*Tel.*), Mayilánchi, Marutónni (*Mal.*), Górante (*Can.*), Méndhi (*Mah.*), Méndi (*Guz.*), Maritondi (*Cing.*), Dán-bin (*Burm.*), Hinie (*Malay*).

197. The leaves of this common Indian shrub, in almost universal use throughout the East for staining the nails, &c., are well worthy of a trial in the treatment of that troublesome and painful affection of the natives called *Burning of the Feet.* For this purpose the fresh leaves should be beaten into a paste with vinegar or lime juice, and applied as a poultice to the soles of the feet. Another plan, which is sometimes more effectual, is to use strong friction with the bruised leaves over the parts. Like all other remedies, however, they not unfrequently fail to afford more than temporary relief; still, from occasionally succeeding, they merit a fair trial.

198. **Leeches.**

Jók (*Hind.*), Jónk (*Duk.*, *Beng.*, *Punj.*), Drik (*Kash.*), Attái (*Tam.*), Attalu, Jela-galu (*Tel.*), Attá (*Mal.*), Jígani (*Can.*), Jala (*Guz.*), Kudallu, Púndal (*Cing.*), Míyon, Minyon (*Burm.*), Lintah (*Malay*).

199. Leeches are procurable, especially during the monsoon, in most parts of India, in the neighbourhood

of tanks and swamps. As they are a valuable resource in many diseases, when properly applied in proper cases, a few preliminary remarks may be acceptable.

200. Leeches vary considerably in size; and their blood-extracting capacity is, as a general rule, in proportion to their size. It has been found that small Leeches will abstract two and a half times, small middle-sized four times, large middle-sized five and a half times, and large ones nearly six times their own weight of blood. Hence, to abstract a certain quantity of blood, a very much larger number of small Leeches is required than of large ones. The middle-sized Leech, from 1½ to 2 inches in length when at rest, is in all cases preferable. The very small Leeches so commonly supplied in India are objectionable on account of the number of bites, the length of time required in their application, and the indefinite small oozing of blood which follows their application, and the difficulty in arresting the flow by pressure. On the other hand, the very large Leech is objectionable from the large gaping wound left by its bite, which often results in an ugly scar; this applies with peculiar force to childhood and infancy.

201. Where only one or two Leeches have to be applied, they may be taken in the hand and held to the spot where it is desired they should bite, but this is a long and tedious process; when several are to be applied, they should be put in a wine-glass, and thus held to the surface till they have all taken.

202. In order to make Leeches bite readily,

thoroughly cleanse the skin with soap and water, and then dry it; this is particularly necessary if a liniment has been previously employed. If they will not bite, one or more of the following plans may be tried:—1. Remove them from the water and keep them for ten minutes in a dry, warm cloth. 2. Smear the skin with cream or sugared milk. 3. Apply a small mustard poultice over the spot. After carefully cleansing with hot water, apply the Leeches. Not only will they bite more readily, but the flow of blood will be far greater than it otherwise would be. 4. Make a small puncture or scratch on the skin, and smear the blood over the surface; this often succeeds when everything else fails. It should also be remembered that the fumes of sulphur, vinegar, or tobacco in a room, will often prevent Leeches from biting at all.

203. To make Leeches bite on particular spots, take a piece of blotting-paper, and make in it as many small holes as there are Leeches, the holes corresponding with the spots on which it is desired to apply the Leeches; they are then to be covered over with a wine-glass or tumbler; the Leeches, finding themselves on a rough surface, creep about till they come to the holes in the paper, when they instantly bite the exposed points of the skin: the blotting-paper is easily removed by being moistened.

204. When Leeches will not drop off naturally, which they generally do in about fifteen minutes or less, or if you wish to remove them, sprinkle them with a little salt or vinegar, or touch them with a piece of onion; the last is an old Bengali practice.

205. To promote the bleeding from Leech-bites, use hot fomentations; to arrest it, apply burnt rag, and make firm pressure with the finger over the bite. A piece of tobacco leaf, or spider's web, or the nap off a hat, sometimes succeeds better than burnt rag. If these fail, try powdered Alum (25), or Sulphate of Copper (116). See also *Hæmorrhage* in Index.

206. If Leeches get into the rectum or nostrils, or any of the other passages, they may be dislodged by using an injection of, or by simply touching them with vinegar or a solution of salt.

207. Leeches should not be applied immediately over a large prominent vein, nor to the eyelids, nor to the bosom of a woman, especially during pregnancy, nor to the loose skin of the penis or scrotum, as the bites in these situations are apt to be followed by infiltration or inflammation.

208. Additional care is necessary in applying Leeches to young children as they bleed so much more freely than adults; they should, when practicable, be placed where a bone is near the surface, so that in case of excessive bleeding pressure may be made against it. Morning is the best time for their application; if put on in the evening, the bites may burst out bleeding whilst the attendants are asleep, and the child die from hæmorrhage; such cases are on record. As a general rule, one Leech is sufficient for each year of a child's age up to six; after that age up to adolescence, the latter number continues to be enough in ordinary cases.

209. *In Fevers attended with much Headache*, Leeches

are very useful, but they should only be applied in the early stages of the disease; when the patient is young and vigorous, four or six Leeches to each temple may be applied, but they sometimes give most relief if put at the nape of the neck, close to the point where the head joins to the spine. *In severe Pain in the Chest or Abdomen occurring during Fevers*, eight or ten Leeches applied immediately over the seat of pain often afford manifest relief.

210. *In severe Headache, or fulness of Head depending upon the stoppage of a discharge of blood from Piles*, Leeches close to the anus frequently afford great relief, but great care is necessary to prevent them creeping up into the rectum. When the *Headache depends upon the sudden stoppage of the Menstrual Discharge*, the Leeches should be applied to the inner part of the thighs.

211. *In Acute Dysentery*, a few Leeches (six to nine) to the verge of the anus are often most serviceable in relieving the pain and straining at stool, and otherwise prove beneficial. The same measure is also of great service in *Congestion of the Liver*, or they may be placed over the region of the liver, but a fewer number afford a greater amount of relief when applied to the verge of the anus.

212. *In all local Inflammations of the Skin, Incipient Abscesses, Boils*, and *in Bruises, Sprains*, and *Blows*, where there is much pain and heat of the part, six or eight Leeches, followed by hot fomentations, tend to relieve the pain and cause the subsidence of inflammatory action.

213. *Obstinate Vomiting* may occasionally be checked by a few Leeches to the pit of the stomach after ordinary means have failed.

214. **Lemon-grass Oil.** The oil obtained by distillation from several species of Andropogon.

Akyá-ghas-ká-aitr (*Hind.*), Hazár-masáleh-ká aatar (*Duk.*), Agya-ghans-tail (*Beng.*), Vásh-anap-pullu-yenney, Karpúra-pullu-yenney (*Tam.*), Nimma-gaddi-núnay (*Tel.*), Vásanap-pulla-enna (*Mal.*), Purvaḷi-hullú-yanne (*Can.*), Lilli-chaya-tél (*Guz.*), Pengrimá-tel (*Cing.*), Sabalen-si (*Burm.*), Miniak Sarie (*Malay*), Iz-khar (*Punj.*), Babber-i-Khát (*Kash.*).

215. Specimens of Lemon-grass Oil met with in India differ somewhat in appearance, but they all partake more or less of the same medical properties, being powerful stimulants whether taken internally or applied externally. The true Lemon-grass Oil is of a pale-sherry colour, transparent, with an extremely pungent taste and a peculiar fragrant lemon-like odour.

216. *In Flatulent Colic and other Spasmodic affections of the Bowels*, a dose of from 3 to 6 drops on sugar or in emulsion often affords great and speedy relief. Thus given it proves effectual in allaying *Obstinate Vomiting.* Even in *that of Cholera* it has been found successful when other remedies have failed, and in these cases it proves additionally serviceable by acting as a stimulant to the system generally; it is

well worthy of a more extended trial in the treatment of this disease. The dose (5 or 6 drops) may be repeated every hour or oftener in severe cases.

217. *In Chronic Rheumatism, Lumbago, Neuralgic Pains, Sprains, and other painful muscular affections,* an embrocation of equal parts of this oil and any bland oil, well rubbed in twice daily, has been found useful in many instances. In old chronic cases it is necessary to use the undiluted oil in order to obtain relief.

218. **Lime.**

Chúnah, Chúna (*Hind.*), Chunnah (*Duk.*), Chún, Chúná (*Beng., Punj., Kash.*), Shunnámbu (*Tam.*), Sunnam (*Tel.*), Núra (*Mal.*), Sunná (*Can.*), Chunná (*Mah.*), Chúno (*Guz.*), Hunu (*Cing.*), Thónphiya (*Burm.*), Kapor (*Malay*).

219. Lime in a medical point of view is of great importance as the basis of LIME WATER, a mild and useful antacid; it is prepared by adding two ounces of Slaked Lime to one gallon of Water, in a stoppered bottle, shaking well for two or three minutes, and then allowing it to stand till the Lime is deposited at the bottom. In cases of emergency, as burns, &c., half an hour is sufficient for this purpose; otherwise it should be allowed to stand for twelve hours at least before being used. It is only the clear water which holds a portion of Lime in solution, which is employed in medicine. It is advisable always to keep a supply ready prepared, as it is useful in many ways, and it will remain good for a long time, if kept in well stop-

pered bottles, so that the air cannot have access to it. The dose for adults is from 1 to 3 ounces twice or thrice daily ; it is best administered in milk.

220. Another form, called the SACCHARATED SOLUTION OF LIME, thought to be better adapted for internal use in the diseases of childhood and infancy, is prepared by carefully mixing together in a mortar one ounce of Slaked Lime and two ounces of powdered White Sugar, and adding this to a pint of Water, as described above. It should be kept in a well stoppered bottle. The dose of the clear water is from 15 to 20 drops or minims in milk twice or thrice daily.

221. *In Acidity of the Stomach, in Heartburn, and in those forms of Indigestion arising from or connected with acidity of the stomach,* Lime Water in doses of 1½ to 2 ounces, is often speedily and permanently effectual. It is particularly useful in indigestion when the urine is scanty and high coloured, and when vomiting and acid eructations are prominent symptoms. It is best given in milk.

222. *In Diarrhœa arising from Acidity* Lime Water frequently proves useful ; it is best given in a solution of gum arabic or other mucilage, and in obstinate cases ten drops of Laudanum with each dose increase its efficacy ; it may also be advantageously combined with Omum water (317). *In Chronic Dysentery* the same treatment sometimes proves useful. Enemas of Lime Water diluted with an equal part of tepid milk or mucilage have also been used with benefit. It is especially adapted for the *Diarrhœa and Vomiting of Infants and young children which result from artificial feeding ;*

in these cases a sixth or a fourth part of Lime Water may be added to each pint of milk. The Saccharated Solution of Lime (220) has also been found of great service in this class of cases.

223. *Obstinate Vomiting* sometimes yields to a few doses of Lime Water in milk, when other more powerful remedies have failed. It is worthy of a trial in the *Vomiting attendant on the advanced stages of Fever;* it has been thought to arrest even the black vomit of yellow fever. It is also a remedy of much value in *Pyrosis or Waterbrash.*

224. *To relieve the distressing Irritation of the Genital Organs* (*Pruritus Pudendi*), bathing the parts well with tepid Lime Water three or four times a-day sometimes affords much relief. *Leucorrhœa and other Vaginal Discharges* have in some instances been mitigated and even cured by the use of vaginal injections of a mixture of 1 part of Lime Water and 2 or 3 of Water.

225. *In Scrofula,* Lime Water in doses of ½ ounce in Milk, three or four times a-day, proves beneficial in some cases; it is thought to be especially adapted for those cases in which abscesses and ulcers are continually forming. To be of service, it requires to be persevered in for some time. *Scrofulous and other Ulcers attended by much discharge* have been found to improve under the use of Lime Water as a local application. For *Syphilitic Ulcers or Chancres,* one of the best applications is a mixture of Lime Water ½ pint, and Calomel 30 grains; this—commonly known as Black Wash—should be kept constantly applied to the part

by means of a piece of lint or rag moistened with it. Many forms of *Skin Disease,* attended with much secretion and with great irritation or burning, are benefited by Lime Water either pure or conjoined with oil (229). *To sore or cracked Nipples* it proves very serviceable. Diluted with an equal part of water or milk it forms a useful injection in *Discharges from the Nose and Ears* occurring in scrofulous and other children.

226. *In Consumption,* Lime Water and milk has been strongly recommended as an ordinary beverage. The same diet-drink has been advised in *Diabetes;* but little dependence is to be placed upon it as a *cure;* it may produce temporary benefit.

227. *In Thread Worm,* enemas of 3 or 4 ounces of Lime Water, repeated two or three times, have sometimes been found sufficient to effect a cure.

228. *In Poisoning by any of the Mineral Acids,* Lime Water given plentifully in milk is an antidote of no mean value, though inferior to some of the other alkalies. It may also be given in *Poisoning by Arsenic.*

229. *To Burns and Scalds* few applications are superior to LIME LINIMENT, composed of equal parts of Lime Water and a bland oil. Olive Oil is generally ordered for this purpose, but Linseed Oil answers just as well, and where this is not at hand Sesamum Oil (338) forms a perfect substitute. When thoroughly shaken together, so as to form a uniform mixture, it should be applied freely over the whole of the burnt surface, and the parts kept covered with rags

constantly wetted with it, for some days if necessary. This Liniment on cotton-wool, applied to the pustules, is said to be effectual in preventing *Pitting in Smallpox.*

230. **The Lime.**—The fresh fruit of Citrus Bergamia, *Risso.*

Límú, Níbú Nínbú (*Hind.*, *Duk.*), Nébu (*Beng.*), Niúmb (*Kash.*), Elumich-cham-pazham (*Tam.*), Nimma-pandu (*Tel.*), Cheru-náranná, Jonakam-náranná (*Mal.*), Nimbo-hannu (*Can.*), Límbu (*Mah.*), Límbu, Nímbu (*Guz.*, *Punj.*), Dehi (*Cing.*), Sámyá-si, Tambiya-sí (*Burm.*), Limowe Nipis (*Malay*).

231. The fresh juice of the Lime is a valuable resource to the Indian practitioner. In *Scurvy* it deservedly ranks highest in our list of remedies, and should be taken to the extent of not less than three ounces twice daily: the addition of sugar increases its efficacy. Should the patient be very debilitated, it may be advantageously combined with tonics, as Infusion of Chiretta (98), or Decoction of Ním Bark (260). Diluted with half its quantity of water it forms an excellent gargle for *Scorbutic and other Ulcerations of the Mouth, and Sponginess of the Gums.* When scurvy appears in a jail or other place where numbers of people are congregated together, the daily use of Lime Juice should be strictly enforced amongst the healthy, as it is one of our best preservatives against an attack of the disease. For other remarks, see Art. *Scurvy*, in Index.

242. *In Smallpox, Measles, Scarlatina, and other forms of Fever*, where there is a hot, dry skin, and much thirst, a very useful refrigerant drink, 'Lemonade,' may be made by pouring a pint of Boiling Water on five or six peeled Limes cut in thin transverse slices. When cool, strain, sweeten to taste, and let the patient drink as plentifully as he likes. In the same class of cases, when the mouth is dry and clammy, sucking a fresh Lime cut in slices is often both agreeable and useful, though when at hand a slice of Pineapple is said to answer the purpose even more effectually. The stringy portion should not be swallowed. *In Diabetes*, weak lemonade is preferable to plain water for allaying the great thirst; like other fluids, in this disease, it is better taken during the intervals between, than at meals.

233. *In cases of Hœmorrhage from the Lungs, Stomach, Bowels, Uterus, Kidneys, or other internal organs*, especially when attended with feverish symptoms, the drink described in the last section, or made somewhat stronger, may be taken with advantage in considerable quantities. The patient should at the same time remain quiet in the recumbent position, and kept as cool as possible.

234. *In Poisoning by Croton Oil Seeds, Castor Oil Seeds, the Physic Nut, and the fresh root of the Bitter Cassava, Mandioc, or Tapioca plant*, almost immediate relief to the purging, vomiting, and other urgent symptoms will be obtained by drinking Lime Juice, 4 or 5 ounces at a time, diluted with an equal quantity of conjee or plain water. It is an antidote

which should always be first tried, because it is generally at hand, and seldom fails to afford more or less relief. A full dose of Castor Oil should be subsequently given.

235. *For relieving the irritation, &c., of Mosquito bites*, the local application of Lime Juice often proves more effectual than anything else. Applied to the surface at nights before going to bed, it is thought also to afford protection from the attacks of mosquitoes.

236. **Moringa, or Horseradish Tree.** Moringa pterygosperma, *Gærtn.*

Shájnah, Ségvá (*Hind.*), Mungé-ká-j*h*ár (*Duk.*), Sojná (*Beng.*), Sohánjná (*Punj.*), Morúnga, Murungai (*Tam.*), Munaga (*Tel.*), Murinna (*Mal.*), Nugge-gidá (*Can.*), Munagá*cha*-jháda (*Mah.*), Murungá (*Cing.*), Dándalon-bin (*Burm.*), Kaylor, Ramoongie (*Malay*).

237. The fresh root of this tree closely resembles in taste, smell, and general appearance, the common Horseradish of Europe, hence its ordinary name amongst Anglo-Indians. There is good reason for supposing that it possesses similar medical properties as a stimulant and diuretic, and in these characters it is worthy of trial in *Dropsical Affections attended with Debility:* it may be given as follows. Take fresh Moringa Root and Mustard Seed, of each, well bruised, one ounce, Boiling Water, one pint; infuse for two hours in a covered vessel and strain. Of this the dose is about one ounce and a half (a wineglassful) thrice

daily. It may also be used as a vehicle for nitre and other more active remedies.

238. *In Hoarseness and Relaxed Sore Throat*, a decoction of Moringa root (or the above infusion) has been found serviceable as a gargle.

239. In the preparation of mustard poultices when it is desired to make them act more speedily or energetically, the addition of the expressed juice of the fresh root, or the scraped root, answers these purposes effectually.

240. **Mudar.** Calotropis procera and C. gigantea, *R. Brown.*

Ák, Ákond, Madár (*Hind.*, *Punj.*), Ák, Ákrá (*Duk.*), Ák, Ákondo (*Beng.*), Ak-a-múl (*Kash.*), Erukku or Erukkam (*Tam.*), Jillédu-chettu, Mándáramu (*Tel.*), Erukka (*Mal.*), Yakkeda-gidá (*Can.*), Ákda-cha-jháda (*Mah.*), Ákda-nu-jháda (*Guz.*), Vára, Vára-gaha (*Cing.*), Mayo-bin (*Burm.*), Ramegu (*Malay*).

241. One or other of the above species of Calotropis is found everywhere in India, and although some doubt exists as to which of them is the Mudar which some years since attained high repute in the treatment of leprosy, they both possess the same medical properties and may be used indiscriminately. The only part employed in medicine is the root-bark; and it is necessary carefully to attend to the subjoined directions for collecting and preparing it for medical use, a disregard of them having been, in some instances, the apparent cause of the failure of the remedy. The

roots should be collected in the months of April and May, from sandy soils, and all particles of sand and dirt having been carefully removed by washing, they should be dried in the open air, without exposure to the s ., until the milky juice contained in them becomes so far dried that it ceases to flow on incisions being made. The bark is then to be carefully removed, dried, reduced to powder, and preserved in well corked bottles. In small doses, from 2 to 5 grains, long continued, its action is that of an alterative tonic; in larger ones, from 30 to 60 grains, for adults, it acts freely as an emetic, and in this character it is regarded by some as one of the best Indian substitutes for Ipecacuanha.

242. *In Leprosy, Constitutional Syphilis, Obstinate Ulcerations, and in Chronic Rheumatism; also in Skin Diseases arising from the abuse of Mercury*, powdered Mudar (*ante*) has been found highly useful in some instances, whilst in others it has altogether failed. The commencing dose is 3 grains, gradually increased to 10 grains or more, thrice daily.

243. *In the Dysentery of Natives* it has been highly spoken of. In the severer class of cases in adults, a large dose, from 20 to 60 grains, may be given at once, in the same manner as Ipecacuanha (see Art. *Dysentery* in Index). In ordinary cases, smaller doses are preferable. For children the dose is 1 or 2 grains for every year of age, three or four times a day. Its effects are said to be very similar to those of Ipecacuanha, like which, it may be given variously combined, as circumstances may require.

244. **Mustard.** The seeds of Sinapis juncea, *Linn.* and other species of Sinapis.

Rái Ráyán (*Hind., Duk.*), Rái (*Benj., Punj.*), Ásúr (*Kash.*), Kadugú (*Tam.*), Áválu (*Tel.*), Katuka (*Mal.*), Sásave (*Can.*), Moharé (*Mah.*), Ráyi (*Guz.*), Abbé (*Cing.*), Munniyén-zi (*Burm.*), Biji Sa-sarvi (*Malay*).

245. English Mustard imported in bottles is procurable in most of the large bazaars, or is met with as an article of domestic economy in the household of almost every European. If not at hand, however, the common country Mustard seed may be substituted, especially in the formation of poultices. For this purpose, however, they require to be thoroughly ground down into the required consistence with a little water. If previously deprived of their fixed oil by expression, their activity is increased. By long keeping they lose much of their pungency; hence fresh seeds should when practicable be employed.

246. With English Mustard at hand you can never be in want of a safe and efficient emetic. A full teaspoonful (piled up) in a tumblerful of warm water, generally produces free vomiting; if it does not, in five or ten minutes it may be repeated, and should this not produce the desired effect, a third dose may be given after a similar interval. Should this fail, then some other emetic may be tried. It is especially indicated in *Drunkenness, Narcotic and other Poisoning, and in all cases where the stomach is overloaded with hard, indigestible food or intoxicating drinks*, when it is desirable

simply to unload the stomach without producing any depressing effect on the system. It is very doubtful whether country Mustard may be safely used as an internal medicine.

247. MUSTARD POULTICES are usually made with the flour of Mustard mixed to the consistence of a poultice with water or vinegar, spread on a piece of stout brown paper or rag, and applied to the skin. A few points require notice :—*a.* Cold water should be used in their preparation; it is a mistake to suppose that hot water or vinegar is better suited for this purpose. *b.* If it be desired to make the poultice act more speedily or strongly, this may be done by adding a small portion of bruised Capsicum or the scraped fresh root of the Moringa tree (239). *c.* For persons of delicate skins, as women and children, it is advisable to place a piece of thin muslin between the poultice and the skin; for the sake of cleanliness also this is desirable. *d.* As a general rule it should be removed when it produces redness of the skin, whether it causes much pain or not. *e.* Some skins are very susceptible to its action; in these cases the poultice should be at once removed if it causes great pain. *f.* If allowed to remain in contact with the skin for twenty or thirty minutes it is apt to act as a blister, which is very undesirable, as the ulcers which result are difficult to heal. *g.* In cases of fever and acute disease, the morning or early part of the day is preferable to the evening for applying a Mustard poultice.

248. *In Apoplexy, Convulsions, Delirium, and violent Headaches occurring during Fevers or Small-pox,* Mustard

poultices to the feet and calves of the legs are often very useful in relieving the affection of the head. Where the patient is able to sit up for the purpose, a Mustard foot bath [an ordinary foot bath, to which is added a handful of Mustard] is even more effectual. The water should be as hot as can be well borne, and the higher the fluid reaches up the leg, the better. In *Delirium Tremens* it should be used every night before bed-time.

249. *In some Head Affections, e. g. the early stages of Insanity, and Delirium Tremens where there is determination of blood to the head, with sleeplessness, restlessness and anxiety*, a plan which has been found effectual in some cases has been to envelope the whole of the legs and lower part of the abdomen in clothes steeped in a mixture of Mustard and hot water, a cold wet towel being at the same time applied round the head. It has a very calming effect, and is occasionally productive of sleep. The Mustard foot bath, described in the last section, is also worthy of a trial, repeated every night before the usual bed-time.

250. *In Dropsy* Mustard occasionally proves useful. It is best administered in the form of Whey, made by boiling half an ounce of the bruised seed in a pint of milk, and straining. This quantity may be given daily in divided doses.

251. *In Cholera, Colic, and Spasms of the Bowels*, when unattended by inflammation, a Mustard poultice placed over the abdomen in many cases affords considerable relief. *Vomiting, especially that accompanying Fevers*, may often be allayed by a Mustard poultice

applied to the pit of the stomach. *In Cholera*, when the patient is very low, the poultice may be placed over the heart, or the left side of the chest.

252. *In Coughs, attended with much difficulty of breathing*, Mustard poultices to the chest often afford relief. They may also be advantageously applied on the back between the shoulder-blades. They may be used for children as well as adults. *Hooping Cough* is occasionally much relieved by Mustard poultices along the spine.

253. *Toothache, Faceache, and Neuralgic Pains of the Head and Face*, are frequently relieved by the application of a Mustard poultice over the seat of pain.

254. **Myrobalans, Chebulic.** The dried fruit of Terminalia Chebula, *Retz.**

Har, Harrá, Pílé-har (*Hind.*), Haldá, Harlá, Pílá-halrá (*Duk.*), Háritakí, Hórá (*Beng.*), Zard-halélá (*Punj.*, *Kash.*), Kadú-káy (*Tam.*), Karak-káya (*Tel.*), Katukká (*Mal.*), Alale-káyi (*Can.*), Hiradá (*Mah.*), Harlé, Pílo-harlé (*Guz.*), Aralu (*Cing.*), Buah Kaduka (*Malay*).

* Mr. W. Martindale, chemist, of New Cavendish Street, London, has forwarded to me a preparation of another kind of Myrobalans, Emblic Myrobalans, the fresh fruit of *Phyllanthus Emblica* (*Linn.*), a common Indian tree, preserved in sugar. The pulp, which has an agreeable taste, is stated by Mr. M. to possess purgative properties in doses of one or two of the preserved fruit. Commenting on this preparation it is stated in the *British Medical Journal* (July 29, 1882, p. 173): 'We have tried it carefully in several cases of habitual constipation, and have no doubt it is a valuable addition to our list of laxatives. . . . It may be eaten at dinner or dessert, and it

255. Chebulic Myrobalans, met with in all the bazaars of India, are of an ovoid shape, about an inch in length, sometimes tapering towards the lower extremity, round or obscurely five or six-sided, more or less furrowed longitudinally, smooth, of a yellowish brown colour, and astringent taste.

256. Myrobalans is a safe and effective aperient, and given to Natives in the following form has been found to act very satisfactorily :—Take of Myrobalans bruised 6, Cinnamon or Cloves bruised 1 drachm, Water or Milk 4 ounces; boil for ten minutes, strain, and set aside till cold. This quantity taken at a draught generally produces on an adult Native three or four copious stools without griping, vomiting, or other ill effects. Youths from twelve to fourteen years require only half the above quantity, or even less. For infants and young children Castor Oil or Senna is preferable as an aperient. It is well adapted for ordinary cases of *Constipation occurring in Natives* and in other states where aperients are required.

257. *Chronic Ulcerations, Ulcerated Wounds, and many Skin Diseases attended with profuse discharge,* often manifestly improve under the use of an oint-

would be absurd to regard it as a medicine. It is most valuable for children.' It should be added that it is only in the fresh state that it possesses aperient properties; in the dried state, as they are commonly met with in Indian bazaars, they are astringent, containing a large proportion of of gallic acid. Their ordinary vernacular names are Ánvulá, Ánvurah (*Hind.*), Ámlá Ánlá (*Beng.*), Nelli-kay, Tóppi (*Tam.*), Ámalakamú (*Tel.*), Nelli-káyi (*Can. Mal.*), Avalá (*Mah.*), Nelli, Nellika (*Cing.*), Zíphiyu-sí (*Burm.*).

ment composed of equal parts of dried Myrobalans and Catechu, both finely powdered, and sufficient ghee or some bland oil to make them into a thick paste: this, spread on a rag, should be applied to the part, and renewed twice daily.

258. **Ním Tree or Margosa.** Azadirachta Indica, *Juss.*

Nínb, Nímb (*Hind.*), Ním (*Duk. Beng. Punj.*), Vémbu, Véppam, Véppa-marum (*Tam.*), Véppa-chettu, Ním-bamu (*Tel.*), Véppa, Aviya-véppa (*Mal.*), Béviná-mará (*Can.*), Límbacha-jháda (*Mah.*), Límbdanu-jháda (*Guz.*), Kohumba, Nímba-gahá (*Cing.*), Tamá-bin, Kamákha (*Burm.*), Dawoon Nambu, Baypay (*Malay*).

258 *b*. The Ním Tree, according to Dr. Pulney Andy (*Madras Jour. of Med. Sci.*, vol. xi. (1867), p. 105), is held in veneration by the Hindús as being dedicated to the goddess Mariathá, the deity which is supposed by them to preside over all epidemics: or rather the epidemics themselves are thought to be visitations of this goddess, in honour of whom the leaves are in common use amongst Hindús, particularly in *Small-pox* epidemics. The leaves are spread on the bed of the patient, fans made of them are used for fanning him, besides which a bunch of them is fixed above the door as a sign of the presence of the goddess in the house. Dr. Pulney Andy was thus led to make trials of the fresh tender young leaves as an internal remedy in fourteen cases, and of these thirteen recovered; but

how far the recoveries were due to the remedy is very problematical. He prescribed about five grains made into a pill, with liquorice powder, and a few drops of water, thrice daily. In the absence of fresh leaves he suggests the use of dried ones in infusion or decoction (ʒi to Water Oi) in doses, for an adult, of one ounce twice or thrice daily. The efficacy of this remedy is open to grave doubts.

259. Ním bark varies much in appearance, according to the size and age of the tree producing it. The bark from the trunk of a tree above three or four years of age is covered with a thick scaly epidermis, and varies in thickness from a quarter to half an inch. That from the smaller branches is smooth, of a dullish purple colour, marked by longitudinal lines of ash-coloured epidermis from one-eighth to one-twelfth of an inch apart. The inner layer of the bark, of a whitish colour in the fresh state, is powerfully bitter, far more so than the outer dark-coloured layer, which, however, possesses a greater amount of astringency. According to the analysis of Mr. Broughton it contains a bitter neutral resin, in which apparently the activity of the remedy resides.

260. Ním bark is a valuable astringent tonic, and when dried and reduced to powder, may be given in doses of one drachm three or four times a day. A better form, however, is a Decoction prepared by boiling two ounces of the bruised inner layer of the bark in a pint and a half of water for a quarter of an hour, and straining whilst hot; of this, when cold, the dose is from 2 to 3 ounces. It, as well as the Powdered

Bark, is a remedy of considerable value in *Ague or Intermittent Fever;* and in these cases it should be given every second hour previous to the time at which the attack is expected to return. It is chiefly adapted for mild, uncomplicated cases, especially in Natives. *For Convalescence after Fevers, General Debility,* and *Loss of Appetite,* the Decoction, in somewhat smaller doses than those mentioned above, proves of great service, and its efficacy is increased and its taste improved by the addition of a few bruised Cloves or a little Cinnamon. As the decoction readily spoils in hot weather, it should be prepared fresh for use when required.

261. *To Indolent and Ill-conditioned Ulcers, especially those of long standing,* a poultice of Ním leaves acts beneficially as a stimulant. It is easily prepared by bruising a sufficient quantity of the fresh leaves with a little tepid water, and applying it, spread on a rag, to the ulcerated surface; should it cause pain and irritation, as it sometimes does, an equal weight of rice flour may be added.

262. Nitre, Saltpetre, Nitrate of Potash.

Shórá (*Hind., Duk., Punj.*), Sórá (*Beng.*), Saféd-shora* (*Kash.*), Pot-luppu (*Tam.*), Peti-luppu, Shúrá-karam (*Tel.*), Veti-uppa (*Mal.*), Pet-luppu (*Can.*), Shóra-mítha (*Mah.*), Sóro-khár (*Guz.*), Pot-lunu, Vedi-lunu (*Cing.*), Yán-zin (*Burm.*), Sundawa (*Malay*).

* In Kashmir the term Shorá means Gunpowder, hence one must speak of White Gunpowder (*Saféd Shorá*), which is the name of Nitre, if it is wished to procure it. (Dr. Aitchison.)

263. Nitre is obtainable in most of the bazaars of India, but often in a very impure state. To fit it for internal use it should be purified by dissolving it in boiling water, removing the scum after the liquid has been allowed to settle, straining the solution through calico and setting aside to crystallise. Pure specimens, which are sometimes met with in large bazaars, should be in white crystalline masses or fragments, colourless, and of a peculiar, cool, saline taste.

264. *In Fever*, when the skin is hot and dry, the tongue parched, the thirst great, and the urine scanty and high-coloured, an excellent refrigerant drink may be made by dissolving two drachms of Nitre in a quart bottle of thin Conjee, and sweetening to the taste with honey or sugar candy. This quantity may be taken daily, in divided doses as an ordinary drink. Tamarind or Lime Juice may be added to improve the flavour if desired. It will be found to moderate the fever, cause some perspiration, and increase the quantity of urine. Should the patient reject the first one or two doses, it should still be persevered in, unless it should manifestly disagree. *In Smallpox, Measles, Influenza,* and *Catarrhal attacks*, the above drink has also been found useful. For children the strength should be reduced one half or more.

265. *For the relief of Headache and Delirium, occurring in the course of Fever*, a very cold and agreeable lotion for the head may be made by dissolving two ounces of Nitre, and an equal quantity of Sal Ammoniac, in a quart bottle full of Water; this should be applied by constant relays of freshly wetted cloths.

266. *In Inflammatory Sore Throat*, a popular remedy, sometimes successful in the early stages, is a small piece of Nitre allowed to dissolve slowly in the mouth.

267. *In Bleeding from the Lungs, Stomach, Uterus, or other internal organs, attended by Fever*, Nitre proves serviceable, though it is not to be relied upon as the sole means of cure. It may be given in doses of ten to fifteen grains, in three ounces of conjee or simple water four or five times a day; the patient at the same time being kept perfectly quiet and cool.

268. *In Asthma*, great relief in many instances results from the inhalation of burning Nitre. For this purpose, dissolve four ounces of the salt in half a pint of boiling water in an open vessel; immerse moderately thick blotting-paper in it for a few minutes, then dry it by exposure in the air or to the fire; when quite dry, cut it in pieces about four inches square, and keep ready for use. Immediately when an attack threatens, burn one, or, if required, two pieces of this paper, so that the fumes may be freely inhaled; but it should not be held too near the face, or the fumes may prove too irritating, and increase rather than diminish the symptoms. The same measure proves very useful in *Spasmodic Coughs*, whether connected with *Chronic Bronchitis* or not. Persons thus afflicted will do well to burn one or two pieces of this NITRE PAPER in the bedroom before retiring to rest at bedtime, care being taken to prevent the too ready escape of the fumes.

269. *In Gonorrhœa,* a solution of a drachm of Nitre in a pint of rice conjee or decoction of Abelmoschus (2) taken freely as a drink, serves to allay the heat on passing urine. Obstinate cases of *Leucorrhœa* sometimes yield to a combination of Nitre (10 grains) and Alum (5 grains) taken thrice daily. It may be advantageously given in conjunction with Infusion of Moringa (237). Nitre has been found to act beneficially as a diuretic in the early stages of *Dropsy.*

270. *In Acute Rheumatism,* Nitre may be given with advantage, commencing with doses of 40 grains, twice daily: this may be gradually increased to 60, 90, up to 120 grains, the vehicle in each case being half a pint of warm rice conjee. The quantity of Nitre may be diminished as the severity of the symptoms subsides. A strong solution of Nitre (three ounces to a pint of water) forms a most soothing application to the swollen and painful joints; cloths saturated with it should be kept constantly applied; the ease which it affords is often very great.

271. **Nutmegs and Mace.** The products of Myristica officinalis (*Linn.*).

Nutmegs.

Jáé-phal (*Hind., Duk., Beng.*), Záfal (*Kash.*), Jádi-káy (*Tam.*), Jájí-kayà (*Tel.*), Játi-ká (*Mal.*), Jaji-káyi (*Can.*), Jái-phal (*Mah., Punj.*), Jáye-phal (*Guz.*), Jádi-ká, Sádi-ká (*Cing.*), Zádi-phu (*Burm.*), Buah-pala (*Malay*).

272. *Mace.*

Jáé-patrí (*Hind.*, *Can.*, *Tel.*, *Guz.*), Jótri (*Beng.*), Jãuntari (*Punj.*), Jõw-watir (*Kash.*), Jádi-pattírí, (*Tam.*, *Mal.*), Vasá-vási (*Cing.*), Zádi-phu-apóén (*Burm.*), Bunga-pala (*Malay*).

273. Nutmegs and Mace, generally procurable in bazaars, are aromatic, stimulant, and carminative, closely allied to Cloves and Cinnamon, for which they may be substituted. Nutmegs in large doses are thought to possess some narcotic properties, hence some care is necessary in their use.

274. THE NATIVE OR COUNTRY NUTMEG, the produce of Myristica Malabarica, *Lam.*, is larger than the officinal Nutmeg, possesses little of its fragrance or its warm aromatic taste, and is very inferior as an internal remedy. Bruised and subjected to boiling, it yields a considerable quantity of a yellowish concrete oil, which, when melted down with a small quantity of any bland oil, is regarded as an excellent application to *Indolent and Ill-conditioned Ulcers*, allaying pain, cleansing the surface, and establishing healthy action. It deserves a trial as an embrocation in *Chronic Rheumatism.*

275. **Opium.** The inspissated juice of Papaver somniferum, *Linn.*

Afyún (*Hind.*), Afím (*Duk.*), Afím, Afín (*Beng.*, *Punj.*, *Kash.*), Abini (*Tam.*), Abhini (*Tel.*) Kasha-kasha-karappá (*Mal.*), Afímu (*Can.*), Afín (*Mah.*), Afím (*Guz.*), Abin (*Cing.*), Bhain, Bhín (*Burm.*), Afíun (*Malay*)

276. Opium is one of the most valuable medicines we possess when properly employed, but as it is very powerful in its operation, it may be productive of great mischief if used without care and caution, or in unsuitable cases.

277. The Opium procurable in the bazaars is always more or less adulterated, hence the quantity procured in one shop is sufficient to procure a good sleep, whilst the same quantity procured at another shop will perhaps producc no sensible effect whatever on the system. This shows the necessity of great caution in its employment.

278. The uncertainty which attends the operation of bazaar Opium leads me to recommend that establishments at out-stations should be always provided with a supply of genuine Smyrna or Turkish Opium imported from Europe. It seems advisable to have it in two forms—*a.* In 1 grain pills, done up ready in an impermeable covering, like those sold by Kirby and others; by keeping it in this form it is always ready for an emergency. *b.* In the form of Tincture, LAUDANUM, which is a very convenient form when small or fractional doses of Opium are required, or when it is desirable to obtain a *speedy* effect. Fifteen minims contain one grain of Opium; this holds good, however, only with recently prepared or carefully preserved laudanum. It should be borne in mind in all hot climates that evaporation of the spirit constituent will take place even in well stoppered bottles, and that in proportion as this evaporation takes place, the strength of the tincture is increased, so that in

long kept Laudanum ten minims, or even less, may contain a grain of Opium. Hence, in using old Laudanum it is advisable to commence with smaller doses than in that recently prepared; the dose can be subsequently altered according to the effect produced or desired.

279. Preparations of Opium should always be kept under lock and key, or they may disappear at a rate which cannot be accounted for by evaporation, or the heat of the climate! Opium in all its forms is a temptation which few Natives have moral courage enough to resist.

280. The preparations of Opium mentioned above should be reserved for internal administration; for external application, where uniformity of strength is of comparatively little consequence, bazaar Opium may be employed, but even here it is desirable that good specimens of the best kinds should be used. A few additional observations on this point may be acceptable.

281. Of the several kinds of Opium met with in India the chief are:—

1. *Patna Garden Opium;* and 2. *Malwa Opium.*—The former, prepared exclusively for medicinal purposes, occurs in square packages of from two to four pounds weight, covered with layers of talc, and further defended by a case of brown wax about half an inch in thickness. It is solid, brittle in the cold season, of a brown colour, and fine smell; it yields a large proportion (7 to 8, or even 10 per cent) of Morphia. Of Malwa Opium there are many varieties;

of these the two principal are, first, that in flat circular cakes, of about a pound and a half in weight, without any exterior covering; dull opaque, blackish brown, externally; internally somewhat darker and soft; odour resembling that of Smyrna Opium, but less powerful, and combined with a slight smoky smell; taste, intensely and permanently bitter: it yields only from 3 to 5 per cent of Morphia. The other, a superior kind of Malwa Opium, occurs in balls or cakes of smaller size, about ten ounces in weight, covered with a coarse dust composed of broken poppy petals; colour internally, dark brown; texture, homogeneous; odour and taste similar to the other variety; it yields from 7 to 8 per cent of Morphia. The other varieties of Indian Opium, the Himalayan or 'Hill Opium,' the Kandeish, the Kutch, &c., are less applicable than the preceding for medicinal purposes, on account of their varying strength. (*Pharm. of India.*)

282. There are some points connected with the use of Opium, which should always be kept in mind:—

a. Some persons are very intolerant to the action of Opium; in these even the smallest dose produces great nervous excitement, violent headache, and vomiting. When this peculiarity is known to exist, the drug should be avoided.

b. Infants and young children bear Opium badly; cases are on record in which three drops of Laudanum have proved fatal to infants. Still, there are diseases of childhood in which it proves valuable, but in these it should not be given except under professional advice or superintendence.

c. It should be avoided as far as possible during pregnancy. Recent experience seems to show that its frequent or habitual use exercises a prejudicial effect on the fœtus.

d. The previous habits of the patient materially influence the effects of this medicine. A confirmed Opium-taker requires a far larger dose to produce a given effect, than one not habituated to it.

e. When the use of Opium is clearly indicated, and the patient from any cause is unable to swallow, it may be given in an enema; in this case a larger dose, a third or even a half larger, is required than when given by mouth.

f. Whenever in doubt as to the advisability of giving Opium, take the safer course, and—avoid it!

For treatment of poisoning by Opium, see Index.

283. There are many diseases as *Rheumatism, Tumours of different kinds, Cancer, Carbuncles* (*Rajah Boils*), *Abscesses,* and *Ulcers connected either with Leprosy, Syphilis or Scrofula,* in which the pain, especially at night, effectually banishes sleep; here Opium is invaluable. An adult may commence with one grain pill or fifteen drops of Laudanum, taken about an hour before the usual bedtime: if this succeeds in procuring sleep it may safely be repeated nightly; if not, the dose may be doubled the second night, and trebled the third night; but it is not advisable to go beyond this quantity except under professional advice. Even these quantities after a week or two's use lose much of their power, and may require to be cautiously increased. When the pains are lessened and the patient

is improving, the quantity of Opium should be decreased gradually, rather than the whole supply left off at once. *To control the Sleeplessness and Restlessness of Delirium Tremens,* Opium given as above may be necessary, but each dose should be combined with four or five grains of Camphor in the form of pill; in fact, Camphor alone in doses of 2 to 3 grains every three or four hours, exercises a most soothing influence, and when this treatment is adopted, the Opium at bedtime may be given alone.

284. *In Spasmodic Affections of the Bowels, violent Colic, and the Passage of Gall Stones,* and when the pain is violent, a full dose of Opium, *e.g.* 20 to 25 drops of Laudanum in a wineglassful of Omum Water, or Infusion of Sweet Flag root (12), often affords speedy relief; should it not do so, however, in half an hour the dose may be repeated, and a third dose after an hour, should the pain continue unabated. At the same time, hot water fomentations, a turpentine stupe, or a mustard poultice, should be applied externally. When the pain has subsided a dose of Castor Oil is advisable, especially when there is reason to suspect that the attack has arisen from the use of crude or indigestible articles of food.

285. *In Cholera* the practice of giving Opium in large and repeated doses, especially in the solid form, in all stages of the disease, is fraught with danger. Administered judiciously at the proper time, and in proper cases, it is capable of doing much good, but its indiscriminate use often produces the worst effects. At the outset of an attack, few remedies are more

useful when combined with Acetate of Lead. (See Index.) Again, it is a valuable adjunct to the 'Calomel treatment' of Dr. Ayre, which consists in giving from one or two grains of Calomel, with from one to five drops of Laudanum, every five, ten, or fifteen minutes, according to the urgency of the symptoms, till the quantity of Laudanum has reached altogether 60 or 80 drops, when it should be discontinued. An essential part of this treatment, which has sometimes proved very effectual, is the free use of cold water as a drink.

286. *For relieving the pain and irritation of the Bladder, caused by the presence of Stone in the Bladder, Gravel, &c.*, no medicine gives more relief than Opium in full doses, as advised in paragraph 284. It proves, however, even more effectual if introduced into the rectum, either in the form of suppository (two grains of Opium with four grains of Soap), or in enema (30 to 40 drops of Laudanum in two ounces of thin conjee water). It may also be given with great benefit *in Irritable states and Painful Affections of the Kidneys.*

287. *In Retention of Urine arising from Spasmodic Stricture of the Urethra*, a hot bath and a full dose of Opium (25 to 30 drops of Laudanum), followed by a dose of Castor Oil, will often suffice to give relief in recent cases of no great severity following a debauch, exposure to wet, &c. The Opium given in an enema of two or three ounces of rice conjee, sometimes succeeds when it fails if given by mouth.

288. *In Diabetes*, Opium occasionally produces the most beneficial results, especially in old cases occurring

in the aged. It requires to be given in full doses and to be persevered in, the effects being carefully watched; the dose diminished, or the remedy left off altogether, if it gives rise to headache or other bad symptoms. It is worthy of remark, however, that persons suffering from this disease will take large doses with impunity.

289. *In many painful Affections of the Uterus* Opium is of the greatest service. Besides being employed in the form of suppository or enema, as mentioned in paragraph 286, Camphorated Opium Liniment (291) warmed, may likewise be rubbed into the loins, or a hot rice poultice sprinkled with Laudanum applied over the lower part of the abdomen. When given internally in these cases it requires to be given in full doses, and it may be advantageously combined with Camphor (73). For the relief of *After-Pains*, 15 or 20 drops of Laudanum in a wineglassful of Camphor julep, or Omum Water, or a little simple conjee, generally affords speedy relief. *In threatened Abortion from a fall, over exertion*, &c., a similar dose of Laudanum, with perfect rest in the recumbent position, may suffice to prevent further mischief; should there be great restlessness or pain, it may be repeated with advantage.

289*a*. *In Dysentery*, Opium in full and repeated doses (one to two grains three or four times a day) was formerly in great repute, but it has fallen into disuse since the Ipecacuanha treatment has been reintroduced; still amongst the Natives it seems, in many cases, to answer better than the latter drug. Even where Ipecacuanha is employed, a preliminary dose of

Laudanum (25 to 30 drops) is often of great service in enabling the stomach to bear it and in preventing its emetic operation. *For the relief of the local pain, bearing down, and straining in this disease*, a small enema (two ounces) of conjee, with 30 to 40 drops of Laudanum in it, affords more relief than anything else. Opium is a valuable adjunct to Catechu and other astringents in the treatment of *Diarrhœa.*

290. *Vomiting* is sometimes speedily relieved by a few drops of Laudanum (5 to 10 drops) in an effervescing draught, or a little Omum Water. It may also be advantageously combined with Infusion of Cloves and other remedies.

291. There are many external or local diseases, including *Chronic Rheumatism, Lumbago*, and other *Muscular and Neuralgic Pains, Spasms*, and *Bruises, Enlarged Glands, Mumps*, &c., in which simple OPIUM LINIMENT, readily made by rubbing down a drachm of bazaar Opium in two ounces of Cocoanut, Sesamum, or other bland Oil, proves very useful. Its efficacy, however, is greatly increased by conjoining it with an equal quantity of Camphor Liniment (68). This, which may be called CAMPHORATED OPIUM LINIMENT, is an excellent application in many painful external affections. It should be well shaken before being used, which it may be night and morning, or oftener if required; care should be taken not to apply it to an abraded or sore surface; it is only adapted for the sound skin, and not even then if the pain is attended with much heat and redness; under these circumstances, cooling lotions (325, 380) are

better adapted. This Camphorated Liniment, well rubbed in along the course of the spine, is occasionally very useful in *Hooping Cough.* For *Stiff Neck,* warm Laudanum rubbed in over the part answers better.

292. *In Ophthalmia attended with great intolerance of light,* great relief may be obtained by fumigating the eye with the vapour of boiling water, to which has been added a teaspoonful of Laudanum, or a couple of grains of Opium. An excellent eyewash in these cases is composed of Laudanum, Vinegar, and Brandy, each one part, and Water four parts. *Toothache,* depending upon a decayed tooth, is often relieved by a grain of Opium put into the hollow of the tooth; the saliva should not be swallowed. *Earache* also frequently yields to a mixture of equal parts of Laudanum and any bland oil, inserted into the outer passage of the ear on a piece of cotton wool; care should be taken not to push it in too far.

293. *To Painful Piles,* where there is much swelling and heat, a very soothing application is a soft rice poultice, the surface of which has been sprinkled with Laudanum, or smeared over with simple Opium Liniment.

294. **Papaw Tree.** Carica Papaya, *Linn.*

Popaiyáh (*Hind.*), Popáí (*Duk.*), Papaiyá (*Beng.*), Pappáyi (*Tam.*), Boppáyí (*Tel., Can.*), Pappáya (*Mal.*), Pópayá (*Mah.*), Papáyi (*Guz.*), Pepolká (*Cing.*), Pimbo-si (*Burm.*), Papaya (*Malay*).

295. The fresh milky juice of the Papaw has been successfully employed in the treatment of *Worms, especially the common Round Worm or Lumbricus.* The juice should be collected as it flows out from incisions made in the unripe fruit; a tablespoonful suffices for a dose for an adult. It should, whilst quite fresh, be mixed with an equal quantity of honey and two ounces of boiling water, and the whole well stirred. When cool, this should be taken as a draught, and two hours subsequently, one ounce of Castor Oil, with half a tablespoonful of Lime Juice. This process should be repeated two days in succession. Half the above dose is sufficient for a child between three and seven years old, and a third, or about a teaspoonful, for a child under three years of age. Should colic follow its use, draughts of sugar and water, or sugar and milk, should be freely given. *In Ringworm* the unripe Papaw fruit, cut in slices and rubbed on the spots, is said by Dr. H. H. Goodeve to be a very simple and efficient remedy.

296. *In Enlargements of the Spleen and Liver* Mr. Evers (*Indian Med. Gazette,* Feb., 1875) reports highly of the value of the milky juice of the unripe Papaw fruit. Of sixty cases treated with it, thirty-nine were cured. He administered it as follows: About a teaspoonful of the fresh juice was thoroughly mixed with an equal quantity of sugar, and the mass made into three boluses, one to be taken morning, noon, and evening. For children a single drop of the juice with sugar was found sufficient. A poultice of the pulp of the unripe fruit was placed in each case over the enlarged organ;

but on this Dr. Evers places little reliance. From 20 to 25 days was the longest period a patient was under treatment. A nutritious and liberal diet to be enforced. It was found notably useful in recent cases. No ill effects—nothing beyond a feeling of heat in the stomach—followed its use. Should there be gastric or intestinal irritation, a small dose of Opium or Henbane may be combined with the juice.

296 *b*. **Pedalium Murex,** *Linn.*

Bará-ghókrú (*Hind.*, *Duk.*, *Beng.*), Ánai-nerunji, Peru-neranji (*Tam.*), Enuga-palléru-mullu, Káítu-nerinjil (*Tel.*), Ána-nerinnil, Káttu-nerinnil (*Mal.*), Ánne-galu-gidá (*Can.*), Hattí-charáttê (*Mah.*), Motto-ghókru (*Guz.*), Ati-naranchi (*Cing.*), Sule-gí (*Burm.*).

297. This small plant, with its yellow flowers and sharp-spined seed vessel, exhaling when bruised the odour of musk, is common on dry sandy localities, especially on the seaboard of most parts of Southern India. The fresh leaves and stems briskly agitated in cold water convert it into a thick mucilage, nearly of the consistency of the white of a raw egg, inodorous and tasteless. An infusion thus prepared is a highly-prized remedy among the people of Southern India in *Gonorrhœa*. For this purpose half a pint of the above infusion is taken every morning for ten days successively; and under its use great relief to the scalding on the passage of urine is afforded, and a cure in many cases effected. It seems well worthy of further trial.

One of its effects, indeed its principal one, is greatly to increase the flow of urine; hence it might prove useful in some forms of *Dropsy.* Water rendered mucilaginous by this plant soon regains its original fluidity; hence the infusion should be freshly prepared each time it is to be administered.

298. **Pepper, Black.** The unripe fruit of Piper nigrum, *Linn.*

Kálí-mirch, Gól-mirch (*Hind., Punj.*), Kálí-mirchí (*Duk.*), Kálá-morich, Gól-morich (*Beng., Punj.*), Martz (*Kash.*), Milagu, Mulagu (*Tam.*), Miriyálu (*Tel.*), Kuru-mulaka (*Mal.*), Menasu (*Can.*), Miré (*Mah.*), Kálo-mirich, Miri (*Guz.*), Kalu-miris (*Cing.*), Náyu-kon (*Burm.*), Lada hitam (*Malay*).

Black pepper, when fresh and of good quality, is a useful stimulant and stomachic in doses of from 10 to 15 grains or more.

299. *In Cholera* the following pills were formerly held in high repute in Bengal. Take of Black Pepper, Assafœtida, and Opium, each 20 grains; beat them well together, and divide into 12 pills; of these one was the dose, repeated in an hour if required. On account of the quantity of Opium they contain, it is inadvisable to continue their use too long (*See* Par. 285). They are chiefly indicated at the very outset of the attack.

300. *For Piles in aged and debilitated persons* the following Confection is often of great service:—Take of Black Pepper in fine powder, 1 ounce; Caraway fruit in fine powder, 1½ ounce; Honey, 7½ ounces. Rub

them well together in a mortar, and give from one to two drachms twice or thrice daily. It proves useful also in the case of old and weak people suffering from *Descent of the Rectum.* An infusion of Black Pepper (2 drachms of bruised Pepper to 1 pint of Boiling Water) forms a useful stimulant gargle in *Relaxed. Sore Throat, and Hoarseness* dependent thereon.

301. **Physic Nut Plant (English).** Jatropha Curcas, *Linn.*

Jangle-arandí (*Hind., Guz.*), Jangli-yarandí (*Duk.*), Erandá-gách, Bon-bhérandá (*Beng.*), Kátt-ámanaku (*Tam.*), Pépalam (*Tel.*), Káttá-vanaka (*Mal.*), Bettada-haralu (*Can.*), Rána-yerandi (*Mah.*), Valendaru, Erandu (*Cing.*), Késu-gi, Simbo-késu (*Burm.*).

302. A common plant in waste places throughout India. The seeds, which in their native state are an acro-narcotic poison, yield on expression about 30 per cent of a pale yellow oil, which in doses of 12 to 15 drops acts as a purgative equal in action to one ounce of Castor Oil, but is far less certain in its operation and causes more griping than the latter, hence it is rarely employed. Its ill effects are corrected by Lime Juice, as in the case of Croton Seeds (Sec. 120). Diluted with a bland oil (1 part to 2 or 3), it forms a useful embrocation in *Chronic Rheumatism.* The leaves locally applied to the breasts, as directed in Sec. 85, are stated notably to *increase the secretion of Milk;* it is worthy of a trial. More important, however, than the

preceding is the alleged power of the fresh juice to *arrest Bleeding or Hæmorrhage from Wounds.* Baboo Udhoy Chand Dutt (*Indian Med. Gazette*, Oct. 1, 1874) details two cases in which a piece of lint, soaked in the juice and locally applied, at once arrested the bleeding; in one of these cases alum, perchloride of iron, &c., had been previously used without effect. He states that it does not cause pain nor act as a caustic, but seems simply to coagulate the blood, and covers the bleeding surface with a tenacious layer. Further evidence of its styptic powers is recorded by Mr. B. Evers (*Indian Med. Gazette*, March, 1875), who furnishes also an interesting account of a pulsating tumour, 'a varicose aneurism,' situated just above the inner ankle, which was cured (?) by the subcutaneous injection of a drachm of this juice. The styptic properties of this agent seem well worthy of further trial.

302 *b*. **Plantago, or Ispaghúl Seed.** The seeds of Plantago Ispaghula, *Roxb.*

Ispaghúl, Isbaghól (*Hind.*), Isapghól (*Duk., Punj.*), Eshopgól (*Beng.*), Ís-mogul (*Kash.*), Ishappukól-viraí, Iskól-virai (*Tam.*), Isapagála-vittulu (*Tel.*), Isabakólu (*Can.*), Isabagóla (*Mah.*), Isápghól (*Guz.*).

303. Ispaghúl seeds, ovate - elliptical, concave, about an eighth of an inch in length, of a greyish colour, yielding to water an abundance of tasteless mucilage, are procurable in most bazaars, and constitute a highly useful demulcent medicine.

304. *In Dysentery and Diarrhœa* they have been long held in well-deserved repute when given, as advised by the late Mr. Twining, of Calcutta. '*In the Chronic Diarrhœa of Europeans,* who have been long resident in India, benefit (he remarks) often follows the use of demulcents followed by mild tonics. For this purpose the Ispaghúl seeds seem to answer better than any other remedy. The dose for an adult is 2½ drachms mixed with half a drachm of powdered sugar candy. The seeds are exhibited whole, and in their passage through the intestines they absorb as much fluid as makes them swell, and by the time they reach the central or lower portions of the canal, they give out a bland mucilage, and in general they continue to possess the same mucilaginous properties until they have passed through the intestines. If the frequency of the dejections be restrained by anodyne enema, and by using only a small quantity of food, the mucilaginous properties of these seeds are most evident. It is said that a slight degree of astringency and some tonic property may be imparted to the seeds by exposing them to a moderate degree of heat, so that they shall be dried and slightly browned. This remedy sometimes cures the protracted diarrhœa of European and Native children after many other remedies have failed.'

305. *In many affections of the Kidneys and Bladder, in Gonorrhœa, &c.,* attended with pain, local irritation and scalding or difficulty in passing urine, the following decoction is likely to prove serviceable :—Take of Isphagúl Seeds bruised, 2 drachms ; Water a pint ;

boil for ten minutes in a covered vessel, and strain. Of this the dose is from 2 to 4 ounces, three or four times daily or oftener.

306. **The Plantain, or Banana Tree.** Musa sapientum, *Linn.*

Kélah-ká-pér (*Hind.*), Mouz-ká-jhár (*Duk.*), Kéla-gáchh (*Beng.*), Kadali (*Tam.*), Kadali, Arati-chettu (*Tel.*), Vázha-marum (*Mal.*), Bálegida (*Can.*), Kéla-jháda (*Mah.*), Kéla-nu-jháda (*Guz.*), Kehal-gahá (*Cing.*), Napiyá-bin (*Burm.*).

307. The Plantain, or Banana-tree, is extensively cultivated throughout the tropical portion of both hemipheres for the sake of its fruit, which forms a valuable article of diet, and in the dried state is of no mean value as an anti-scorbutic (See Art. *Scurvy* in Index). It is mentioned in this place chiefly on account of its leaves, which, when young and tender, are of a beautifully fine texture, and may be utilised with great advantage in medical and surgical practice.

a. As a dressing for blistered surfaces, for which purpose they are admirably adapted in hot climates, where Spermaceti Ointment, usually employed in European practice, rapidly becomes rancid, and consequently irritant. After the removal of a blister a piece of plantain leaf of the required size, smeared with any bland oil, should be applied to the denuded surface and kept in its place by means of a bandage. The first sensation it occasions is peculiarly cooling and soothing, and the blistered surface generally heals satisfactorily in four or five days. For the first two days the upper smooth surface is placed next to the skin, and subsequently the under side, until the healing process is complete. It should be changed twice daily, or oftener if required.

b. As a substitute for India Rubber or Gutta Percha Tissue in the water-dressing of Wounds and Ulcers. The younger the leaf, the better is it suited for this purpose. Two points require attention: 1, the piece used should be sufficiently large to cover or envelope the whole part; and, 2, it should be carefully kept in its place by bandages, &c. If properly applied, evaporation of any subjacent fluid is effectually prevented.

c. As a shade for the eyes in Ophthalmia and other Diseases of the Eye, no manufactured shade is superior to it; the older and greener leaves answer best for this purpose.

308. **Plumbago rosea,** *Linn.*

Lál-chíta, Lál-chítarak (*Hind.*), Lál-chitarmúl (*Duk.*), Rakto-chitá (*Beng.*), Chitra (*Punj.*), Shitranj (*Kash.*), Shivappu-chittira-múlam, Kodi-múli (*Tam.*), Erra-chitra-múlam (*Tel.*), Chenti-kotuvéli (*Mal.*), Kempu-chitra-múlá (*Can.*), Támbada-chitramúla (*Mah.*), Ratnitúl (*Cing.*), Kin-khen-ní (*Burm.*), Chiraka-merah (*Malay*).

309. The root of this plant, common in gardens throughtout India, is of great value as a means of raising a blister when other articles of the same class are not available. For this purpose take the fresh bark of the root and rub it into a paste with water

and a little rice flour; spread this on a piece of rag and apply it to the surface; in about five minutes it begins to give pain, which increases in severity for about half an hour, when it may be removed: a rice poultice may then be applied over the part, and within twelve or eighteen hours a large uniform blister will be found to have formed. The fluid having been let out, it may be dressed with plantain leaf, in the usual way. The chief objection to the use of a Plumbago blister is the great pain it occasions, hence it should only be used when other blistering agents are not at hand, and a blister is an immediate necessity.

310. **Pomegranate Tree.** Punica Granatum, *Linn.* Anár-ká-pér (*Hind.*), Anár-ká-jhár (*Duk.*), Dálim-gásh (*Beng.*), Dhãun (*Kash.*), Mádalai-chedi (*Tam.*), Dálimba, Dádima-chettu (*Tel.*), Máta-lam-chetti (*Mal.*), Dálimbe-gidá (*Can.*), Dálimba-jháda (*Mah.*), Dádam-nujháda (*Guz.*), Delun-gahá (*Cing.*), Salé-bin, or Talí-bin (*Burm.*), Dalima (*Malay*).

311. Two parts of the Pomegranate tree, common in gardens and elsewhere throughout India, are employed medicinally, viz., the Rind of the Fruit and the Bark of the Root or Root-bark.

312. *In Diarrhœa and the advanced stages of Dysentery*, the rind of the fruit is a valuable astringent. It is best given in Decoction prepared by boiling in a covered vessel, 2 ounces of the bruised Dried Rind, and 2 drachms of bruised Cloves or Cinnamon in a

pint of Water for fifteen minutes and straining. Of this, when cold, the dose is 1½ ounces three or four times a day; in obstinate cases, five drops of Laudanum may be added to each dose. It is said to be especially useful in the *Diarrhœa of Natives.*

313. *In Relaxed Sore Throat* the above decoction, with the addition of a drachm of Alum to the pint, is a very useful gargle, and it also forms a good astringent injection in *Vaginal Discharges;* in these cases the cloves or cinnamon should be omitted.

314. *For Tape Worm* the Root-bark is a remedy of established value given as follows: Take of the fresh Bark sliced, 2 ounces; Water, 2 pints; boil to 1 pint and strain. Of this, two ounces should be taken fasting, early in the morning, and repeated every half-hour, until four doses have been taken. This should be followed by an aperient (1 ounce of Castor Oil), and the worm will generally be expelled within twelve hours. The Root-bark of the male tree is supposed to possess the greatest power in these cases.

315. **Ptychotīs, Ajwain or Omum Seeds.** The fruit of Carum (Ptychotis) Ajowan, *D.C.*

Ajváyan (*Hind.*), Ajvain, Ajván (*Beng.*), Ajván (*Duk.*), Ajwain (*Punj.*), Jáwind (*Kash.*), O'mam, or O'mum (*Tam.*), Omamu, Vámamu (*Tel.*), Hómam, Ayamód-kam (*Mal.*), Vóma (*Can.*), Vóvá, Vóva-sádá (*Mah.*), Ajwán (*Guz.*), Oman, Assamodagam (*Cing.*), Samhún (*Burm.*), Lavinjularmisi (*Malay*).

316. These small, pungent, aromatic seeds rank

deservedly high in the list of native remedies; they are considered to combine the stimulant quality of capsicum or mustard with the bitter property of chiretta, and the antispasmodic virtues of assafœtida. This remedy, Dr. Bidie remarks, in moderate quantities increases the flow of saliva, augments the secretion of gastric juice, and acts as a stimulant, carminative and tonic. As a topical remedy it may be used with advantage along with astringents in cases of *Relaxed Sore Throat.* For disguising the taste of disagreeable drugs and obviating their tendency to cause nausea and griping, he adds, that he knows no remedy of equal power. Testimony of a similar character is borne by Mr. J. J. Wood and others, and no room is left to doubt the value of this medicine.

317. The Natives employ the crude seeds in doses of about a dessert spoonful with the addition of a little salt; this is chewed and washed down with draughts of water. They also employ them in decoction, but this is objectionable, as heat dissipates the essential oil, in which the virtues of the seeds reside. A far better form is the Distilled Water, OMUM WATER,* which is procurable in all the large towns in India, being a very popular remedy with the Native and East Indian portion of the community. Where, however, it is not purchaseable it can be readily prepared by any Native who has a common country still; in this case care

* Aarqe-ajván (*Hind. et Duk.*), Ajwain-ka-arak (*Punj.*) Jawind-húnd-arak (*Kash.*), Óman-tí-nír (*Tam.*), Ómam-drávakam (*Tel.*). It is also sold under the name of 'Sison Cordial.' Every Indian domestic medicine chest should contain a good supply of this useful preparation.

should be taken that the right proportions be used—3lbs. of the bruised seeds to six quart bottles of water, and distil over four. In order to prevent the seeds touching the bottom or side of the boiler, and thus by becoming charred communicating a burnt flavour to the water, they should be tied up in a bag or cloth of loose texture, and suspended in the centre of the water. The dose is from 1 to 2 ounces, repeated as circumstances may require; that for a child ranges from a tea spoonful to a table spoonful, according to age. The Distilled Oil is also an excellent form of administration in doses of 1 to 3 drops on sugar, or made into an emulsion with Gum Arabic.

318. In some forms of *Dyspepsia, in the Vomiting, Griping or Diarrhœa arising from errors of diet; in simple Flatulence and even Tympanites; in Faintness and Exhaustion; in Spasmodic Affection of the Bowels, in Choleraic Diarrhœa, in certain cases of Colic; and in Hysteria,* it has been found, even when given alone, pre-eminently useful (Wood). *It is especially adapted for the Diarrhœa and Flatulent Colic of Children.*

319. *In Cholera* much reliance is placed by the natives and Anglo Indians on Omum Water, and although it appears to have no claim to the character of a specific in this disease which popular opinion assigns to it, there can be little doubt that it exercises considerable power, especially in the early stage, of checking the diarrhœa and vomiting, and at the same time of stimulating the system. It is not to be trusted to alone, but forms an admirable adjunct to other remedies.

320. *In Habitual Drunkenness, Dipsomania,* Omum seems worthy of trial. On this point Mr. Wood observes, 'On account of its biting or pungent, yet pleasant taste, and the sensation of warmth it creates in the stomach, it has been constantly recommended of late years to those afflicted with the desire for alcoholic drinks. It does not, of course, intoxicate, but it is no mean substitute for the ordinary stimulant, in removing almost immediately the sensation of "gnawing" or "sinking at the pit of the stomach," which the frequent use of spirits so invariably brings on. And I have been assured that it has been the means of rescuing many otherwise sensible and useful men from slavery to the habit of spirit drinking.'

321. **Rice.** The husked seed of Oryza sativa, *Linn.*

Chával (*Hind.*), Chánval (*Duk.*), Chál, Chánvol (*Beng.*), Chánwal (*Punj.*), Thormúd (*Kash.*), Arishi (*Tam.*), Biyyam (*Tel.*), Ari (*Mal.*), Akkí (*Can.*), Tándúla (*Mah.*), Chókha (*Guz.*), Hál (*Cing.*), Sán, Chán (*Burm.*), Bras (*Malay*).

322. Rice may be utilised in the following ways in the treatment of disease :—

a. In the form of Decoction—'CONJEE WATER,' as it is commonly called, prepared by boiling one ounce of cleansed Rice in a quart of Water for twenty minutes, straining, and flavouring with Sugar, and with Lime Juice if desired, to taste. This forms an excellent drink in *Fevers, Smallpox, Measles, Scarlet Fever and Inflammations of all kinds,* also in *Gonorrhœa,* and other cases where there is *pain and difficulty in passing Urine.*

b. In the form of Powder—RICE FLOUR; this dusted thickly over the surface forms a very cooling and soothing application in *Smallpox, Measles, Erysipelas, Prickly Heat,* and other *Inflammatory Affections of the Skin.* It is pleasant to the patient's feelings, and allays heat and irritation. *To Burns and Scalds,* Rice Flour is an excellent application: it should be used as soon as possible after the occurrence of the injury, and it should be dusted thickly over the whole of the burnt surface, so as to absorb any discharge that may be present, and at the same time exclude the air as far as possible. If in a few days this becomes hardened and irritating, a warm Rice poultice should be applied, so as to soften it and allow its easy removal; the surface should then be dressed with Lime Liniment (229), or Resin Ointment (372).

c. In the form of Poultice.—RICE POULTICE.—To prepare this, place a sufficiency of Rice Flour in an open vessel over the fire, gradually add Water, and stir until the mass has the required consistence. A more ready mode is to place the Rice Flour in a basin, and then gradually to add Boiling Water, constantly stirring it, as above. A piece of cloth of the required size being ready at hand, the poultice should be smoothly spread on it, to the thickness of from a quarter to half an inch, and applied over the affected part. In most cases it is advisable before applying it, to smear the surface of the poultice with a bland oil; this renders it more soothing and keeps it longer soft.

and moist. A rice poultice requires changing twice or even thrice daily. It is an excellent application to *Abscesses, Boils, Buboes, Ulcers,* and *other local inflammatory affections, Inflamed Piles,* &c. *In Chronic Bronchitis and other Chronic Coughs* considerable relief often results from the application of a large soft Rice Poultice placed over the chest at bedtime, and allowed to remain on all night; another may also be advantageously placed on the back between the shoulder-blades. The efficacy of these poultices is in many cases increased by the addition of a little Mustard Flour (1 part to 3 or 4 of Rice Flour), so as to produce a slight redness of the skin; or the surface of the poultice may be smeared over with Oil of Turpentine.

323. Sal **Ammoniac.** Hydrochlorate of Ammonia, Chloride of Ammonium.

> Nousádar (*Hind.*), Nouságar (*Duk.*), Nosházgar (*Beng.*), Charám, Navá-charám (*Tam.*), Navá-charám, Nava-ságaram (*Tel.*), Nava-sáram (*Mal.*), Navá-ságára (*Can.*), Nav-sága (*Guz.*), Navá-cháram (*Cing.*), Zavasa (*Burm.*), Namu-charum (*Malay*), Nãusbádar (*Punj.*), Nausadan (*Kash*).

324. Sal Ammoniac, procurable in most Indian bazaars, is generally very impure; occurring in thick translucent cakes or masses of a dirty white or brownish colour, inodorous, of a bitter, acrid taste. To fit it for medical use, it should be dissolved in boiling water, strained through calico, and the clear

solution exposed in an open vessel to crystallize. The crystals and white residuum should be collected and kept in bottles for use. Thus prepared, it proves valuable in many affections. Its nauseous taste, which is a great objection to its use, is completely covered by the addition of a small quantity of liquorice.

325. *Milk Abscesses* occurring after confinements and in nursing mothers may often be arrested, if at an early stage, before matter forms, the breast be kept constantly wet by means of rags saturated with a lotion composed of one drachm of Sal Ammoniac, one ounce of Arrack, and a pint of Rose Water. It also proves useful in removing any hardness which may remain after the abscess has burst. It is also sometimes successful in arresting *Abscesses in other parts of the body*, when applied at an early stage before matter has formed.

326. *In Tic Douloureux and Rheumatic Face Ache*, Sal Ammoniac occasionally proves very useful. Two drachms in six ounces of water should be taken in divided doses ($1\frac{1}{2}$ ounce for a dose), every four hours, till relief is obtained; if the pain does not yield after the four doses, no benefit can be expected from persevering with it. *Other forms of Neuralgia*, as *Sciatica* and *Lumbago*, have also been found to yield to it, when administered early in the attack.

327. *In Chronic Rheumatism, especially when the muscles are mainly affected*, Sal Ammoniac, in doses of 15 to 24 grains, with infusion of Country Sarsaparilla (163), proves highly serviceable; but it is even more effectual in relieving those *Muscular pains of the*

Chest and other parts of the trunk so often met with in the over-worked and under-fed portion of the working classes in large cities. In these cases it requires to be persevered in for some time.

328. *Hysterical, Nervous, and Bilious Head Aches* are often greatly benefited, or disappear altogether, under the use of this salt in doses of 10 to 20 grains twice or thrice daily, dissolved in Camphor Julep. The earlier in the attack it is given, the greater are the chances of its proving effectual.

329. *In Chronic Coughs, especially in those of old age,* a mixture of a drachm of Sal Ammoniac, two ounces of Syrup of Country Liquorice (6), and four ounces of Water, in doses of one ounce five or six times a-day, occasionally proves serviceable. In doses of from 1 to 5 grains, according to the age of the child, conjoined with a few grains of powdered Cinnamon, it has been found useful in *Hooping Cough;* it is inferior in efficacy to Alum, but may be commenced with safety and advantage at a much earlier period in the attack.

330. *In Hæmorrhage from the Lungs, Stomach, and other internal organs,* it is worthy of a trial if other more effectual agents are not at hand. In these cases, two drachms should be dissolved in a pint of Conjee Water, and a wineglassful given every second or third hour, according to the severity of the case. The patient should be kept quiet, cool, and in the recumbent posture.

331. *In Jaundice,* especially when it comes on suddenly, after a great mental shock, or after exposure, a few doses of Sal Ammoniac (20 grains every four

hours) have often a marked effect. *In Hepatitis and Abscess of the Liver*, Dr. W. Stewart, after considerable experience in its use, regards this salt almost as a specific, and he pronounces it very serviceable in *all cases of Liver Disease*, whether depending on organic change or on functional derangement. The proper period for its exhibition is after the abatement of acute symptoms, and when diaphoresis (sweating) has been freely established, and it should then be administered in doses of 20 grains night and morning. The evidence he adduces in support of his views is very strong. He also speaks highly of its efficacy in *Chronic Dysentery*, and advises its continued use for some time after the disappearance of acute symptoms. (*Madras Journ. of Med. Science*, 1870, and Feb., March, and Dec., 1872.) *In Dropsy*, especially in that connected with disease of the liver, or in that following fevers, it may be administered with advantage in the same doses, conjoined with Infusion of Moringa (237), or Decoction of Asteracantha (39).

332. *For Bruises, Strains, Rheumatic Swellings, Enlarged Glands, Indolent Buboes, Swollen Joints, Boils,* &c., and *local Inflammations of the Skin* generally, a solution of this salt in *hot* water (2 drachms to a pint), kept to the parts for a few hours, proves useful, not only relieving the pain, but reducing the swelling. It is also thought to be more effectual than anything else in removing the discoloration consequent on bruises and sprains. This has been noticed especially with reference to blows on the eye (*Black Eye*). It is an important ingredient in the Cold Lotion described in Sect. 265.

333. **Sandal-wood Oil.** The oil obtained by the distillation of Sandal Wood, Santalum album, *Linn.*

Sandal-ká-aitr (*Hind.*), Sandal *vel* Chandan-ká-tél (*Duk.*, *Punj.*), Safed-chandnúk-til (*Kash.*), Sandal-ká-tel (*Beng.*), Shandanam-talium (*Tam.*), Miniak Chandana (*Malay*).

334. Sandal Wood Oil is sold commonly in the bazaars, being a favourite native perfume. It has been successfully employed in the treatment of *Gonorrhœa.* Dr. Aitchison strongly recommends commencing with five-drop doses, each dose to be made up separately, and the oil mixed in the fluid it is to accompany with the aid of a drop or two of Liquor Potassæ. It is an excellent remedy, he adds, but must be used with *great care,* as it is apt to produce baneful effects on the kidneys if given in too large doses. It is of great importance to use only good or pure oil: hence it should be procured, if possible, direct from the manufacturer. Much that is sold in the bazaars is adulterated or of inferior quality. It seems well worthy of trial in cases of obstinate *Gleet.* It is best given in a little Omum Water or Infusion of Ginger.

335. **Senna.** The leaves of Cassia lanceolata, *Forsk.*, and other species. Indian or Tinnevelly Senna.

Saná, Hindí-saná-ká-pát (*Hind.*), Nát-kí-saná (*Duk.*), Són-pát, Shín-pát (*Beng.*), Sanna-mákhí (*Punj.*), Berg-i-sanna (*Kash.*), Nilá-virai, Níla-vakái

(*Tam.*), Néla-tangédu (*Tel.*), Níla-váká (*Mal.*), Nelá-varíke (*Can.*), Sana-kola, Nil-ávari (*Cing.*), Puve-kain-yoe (*Burm.*), Sunna Maki (*Malay*).

336. The imported Senna met with in the bazaars is usually of very inferior quality, consisting of broken pieces of old leaves, pieces of stem, and other rubbish. That grown in India, especially in Tinnevelly, is preferable to that imported from Arabia, which is called *Sana-Mukhí*, or *Mecca Senna*. The leaves should be unbroken, clean, brittle, pale green, or yellow, with a heavyish smell. It is a good safe aperient, and may be given as follows: Take of Senna leaves, one ounce; of bruised Ginger and Cloves, each half a drachm; Boiling Water, ten ounces. Let it stand for one hour, and strain. This is a good aperient in all cases of *Constipation*, in doses of one and a half to two ounces; half this quantity, or less, is required for children, according to age. A simple infusion of Senna leaves, of the above strength, if taken hot with the addition of milk and sugar, can hardly be distinguished from ordinary tea. In this manner it is easily administered to children, and will be borne by the most delicate stomachs. As a general rule, Castor Oil is preferable as an aperient for infants.

337. **Sesamum, Jinjili,** or **Til Oil.** The expressed oil of the seeds of Sesamum Indicum, *Linn.**

* This plant (*Sesamum Indicum, Linn.*) is cultivated throughout India and other tropical lands for the sake of its oil-yielding seeds. The leaves, which abound in mucilage, have attained some repute in bowel affections, and Mr. B. Evers (*Indian Med.*

Til-ká-tél, Míthá-tél (*Hind.*, *Punj.*), Mittá-tél (*Duk.*), Nal-enney (*Tam.*), Manchi-núne (*Tel.*), Nall-enná ((*Mal.*), Valle-yanne (*Can.*), Chokhóta-téla (*Mah.*), Mítho-tél (*Guz.*), Talla-tel (*Cing.*), Télmúk-tíl (*Kash.*), Nahu-sí (*Burm.*), Miniak bijan (*Malay*).

338. Til or Jingili Oil, met with in all bazaars throughout India, is quite equal, when properly prepared, to Olive Oil for medicinal and pharmaceutical purposes. It is advisable always to keep a small stock of it on hand for cases of emergency, such as burns, &c., when Lime Liniment (229) may be required. As a dressing for *Ulcers*, *Suppurating Wounds*, 'oil dressing' has been successfully applied in Bombay; it consists of the continuous application of a

Gazette, March, 1875) made trials with them in sixteen cases of *Dysentery*. Recovery followed in each case, but they were all of a mild type, and though the remedy acted as a demulcent, it did not appear to exercise any specific influence on the disease; besides, as Opium had to be conjoined with it to control the turesmus, the benefit may have been due as much, if not more, to the opiate as to the mucilage. It is evidently a remedy of very secondary value, and inferior to Ispaghúl Seeds (304). The seeds have powerfully emmenagogue properties assigned to them, and it is believed by the Natives and Anglo-Indians that, if taken in large quantities, they are capable of producing abortion. In *Amenorrhœa* the employment of a warm hip bath containing a handful of the bruised seeds has been reported on good authority to be an efficient mode of treatment. It seems worthy of further trial. In three cases of *Dysmenorhœa* (*Painful Menstruation*) Mr. B. Evers (*op. cit.*) administered with benefit the powdered seeds in ten-grain doses three or four times daily. At the same time he employed the hip bath containing the bruised seeds as mentioned above.

pledget of common country cloth or rag saturated with pure Sesamum Oil to the affected part. It is thought to be superior to any other simple dressing, particularly during the hot season. *In Leprosy* Dr. Hilson has conclusively shown that great and manifest benefit, though it may be temporary, results from diligent frictions of the body with this oil (see Sect. 161).

339. **Sulphur.**

Gañdak, Gandhak (*Hind.*, *Duk.*, *Mah.*, *Guz.*, *Punj.*, *Kash.*), Gandrok (*Beng.*), Gandakam, Gandhakam (*Tam.*, *Tel.*, *Mal.*; *Cing.*), Gandhaká (*Can.*), Kán (*Burm.*), Blerang (*Malay*).

340. Several kinds of Sulphur are met with in the bazaars, but as their composition is unknown, and some of them are reputed to contain a large proportion of Arsenic, they are unsuited for internal administration; the better and purer kinds, however, may be safely employed as external applications.

341. As a remedy for *Itch*, SULPHUR OINTMENT holds a high place. One part of finely-powdered, or Sublimed Sulphur to six of Lard, Kokum Butter or any bland Oil, is sufficiently strong for ordinary cases. After cleansing the parts with soap and hot water, the ointment should be thoroughly well rubbed in for fifteen or twenty minutes, till the pustules are all broken. Its use should be confined to the hands and wrists and other parts affected; no good is obtained from applying it extensively over the whole surface of the body, as is often done. It is best rubbed in at

might, before going to bed, allowing it to remain on the whole night, and then washing it off in the morning with soap and hot water. This process may be repeated every night till a cure is effected, which will be the case after three or four applications, provided the ointment is properly rubbed in. The patient should not resume the clothes he wore previously until they have been subjected to the process of *boiling*, a temperature of 212° F. being necessary for the destruction of the acarus, on the presence of which the disease depends. Simply washing the clothes in hot water will not destroy the germ of infection.

342. Some other forms of *Chronic Skin Disease in Natives* improve under the use of Sulphur Ointment, described in the last section; or, better still, of 'Balsam of Sulphur' so called, which is simply a solution of sulphur in warm Olive or Sesamum Oil.

343. *In Chronic Rheumatism* a liniment, composed of two ounces of powdered or Sublimed Sulphur, and a pint of Ním Oil, well rubbed in twice daily, has been used with great benefit in many cases. Relief sometimes follows the practice of dusting the affected part with Flour of Sulphur at bedtime, enveloping it in flannel, and covering the whole with plantain-leaf to prevent the escape of the fumes.

344. *In Piles* few medicines afford more relief to the distressing local symptoms than a mixture of equal parts of Sublimed Sulphur and Cream of Tartar; of this a tea spoonful should be taken in milk once or twice daily, so as to keep the bowels gently open. Should this quantity, however, operate too powerfully

on the bowels, the dose should be diminished. The ingredients for this powder should be procured from a regular chemist. The same treatment appears to act beneficially in *Chronic Dysentery.* It is likewise well adapted for *Habitual Constipation*, especially when occurring in persons subject to piles. It is well to bear in mind that in all cases where Sulphur is administered internally, it communicates to the stools a peculiarly disagreeable odour of sulphuretted hydrogen.

345. **Tamarinds.** The Fruit of Tamarindus Indicus, *Linn.*

Anblí (*Hind.*), Amlí, Amlí-ká-bót (*Duk.*), Imlí (*Punj.*), Tamar-i-hind (*Kash.*), Téntúul, Tintúrí, Ámlí (*Beng.*), Puliyam-pazham (*Tam.*, *Mal.*), Chinta-pandu (*Tel.*), Chinch (*Mah.*), Hunashí-hannu (*Can.*), Ámblí (*Guz.*), Siyambula (*Cing.*), Magi (*Burm.*), Assam-java (*Malay*).

346. The pulp of the fruit, of a reddish brown colour and acid saccharine taste, is laxative and refrigerant, and made into sherbet with water or milk (in the proportion of one ounce of the pulp to one pint of fluid) forms an agreeable and useful drink in *Febrile and Inflammatory Affections.* The only objection to it in some cases is (in others this is an advantage) that it is apt to act on the bowels as a laxative. In the absence of limes or lemons, Tamarind pulp may be given with great advantage in *Scurvy,* both as a preventive and as a curative, but it requires to be discon-

tinued if it cause griping and diarrhœa; otherwise it is a valuable antiscorbutic, and as such may be taken on board ship, or form a portion of daily rations in jails, &c.

347. **Telini Fly, Mylabris Cichorii** (*Fabr.*).

Télní, Télní-makkhí (*Hind.*), Zírangí, Bad-bó-kí-zírangí (*Duk.*), Pinsttarin-í (*Tam.*), Blishtering-ígelu (*Tel.*).

348. This insect is of common occurrence throughout India; it has the following characters:—About an inch in length and the third of an inch broad; the elytra, or wing-cases, of an obscure yellow, with three large somewhat zig-zag transverse black bands; the first band is interrupted and sometimes reduced to three or four spots. There are met with in various parts of India other allied species, which differ more or less from the above description, but they all partake of the same irritant and vesicant properties, the active principle being the same with that of the officinal Cantharides, viz., Cantharidine. It is apparently a complete substitute for the European article as a vesicant, provided that due care is taken in its preparation, &c. The best season for collecting the insects is just previous to the setting in of the monsoon, in the early morning or evening; they should be killed by the steam of boiling vinegar, thoroughly dried in the sun, and preserved in well stoppered bottles.

349. Its principal use is as a blistering agent, and

for this purpose it is used in the form of plaster,* prepared as follows:—Take Telini Fly, finely powdered; White or Black Dammar, Bees-wax, and Suet, of each two ounces; liquefy the three latter with a gentle heat, then remove from the fire and sprinkle in the Telini; mix the whole thoroughly, and continue to stir the mixture while it is allowed to cool.

350. *Remarks on the Use of Blisters.*—Blisters are of great value in many cases, but unless used with care and discrimination they may do more harm than good. Thus a blister applied at the outset or during the acute stage of inflammation will increase the mischief, whereas in the advanced stages its action may prove in the highest degree beneficial. During pregnancy a blister to the chest has been known to induce premature labour, retention of urine, &c., and applied to a person suffering from scurvy it is apt to induce troublesome ulceration. To prevent gangrene, which has occasionally resulted from a blister, especially in children, it is advisable not to allow it to remain on more than four or five hours; then to remove it and apply a warm rice poultice. In infants a thin piece

* In consequence of the difficulty of preparing this, and the uncertainty of its strength, I would advise that every establishment should be provided with a supply of officinal Blistering Liquid of the British Pharmacopœia; this only requires to be applied for two or three minutes with a camel's hair brush, allowed to dry on, and then covered with a warm rice poultice; in the course of a few hours the blister will be found to have risen. The Liquid prepared in India from the Telini Fly is quite equal in power to the European article prepared with Cantharides or Spanish Fly.

of muslin should be placed between the skin and the plaster. If strangury follow its use, the patient should drink plentifully of decoction of Abelmoschus (2), Rice Conjee (322), or other demulcents, avoiding those of an oleaginous nature. After the fluid has been let out, which is easily done by snipping the raised cuticle in two or three places with a pair of sharp-pointed scissors, the blistered surface should be dressed with plantain leaf, as directed in paragraph 307*a*.

351. **Tinospora cordifolia**, *Miers.*, **Gulancha.**

Gulanchá, Gul-bél (*Hind.*), Gul-bél (*Duk.*), Gul-lanchá (*Beng.*), Giló, Gúlanch (*Punj.*), Bekh-gilló (*Kash.*), Shindi-kodi (*Tam.*), Tippa-tíge, Gadúchi (*Tel.*), Amruta, Chitr-amruta (*Mal.*), Amruta-balli (*Can.*), Gula-vélí (*Mah.*), Gul-vél (*Guz.*), Rasa-kinda (*Cing.*), Sinza-manné, Singomoné (*Burm.*), Piturali, Akar-sarimtooro (*Malay*).

351*b*. This twining shrub is common in most parts of India. The root and stems, which are the parts employed in medicine, should be collected in the hot season when the bitter principle is most abundant and concentrated. As met with in the bazaars it consists of dried transverse segments of a woody stem, varying in diameter from one quarter of an inch to two inches, and from half an inch to two inches in length; they have a shrunken appearance, and are covered with a smooth shrivelled bark, some of the pieces being marked on their surface with warty prominences; inodorous, of a very bitter taste.

352. Gulancha is a very useful tonic, and is best given in Infusion; one ounce of the bruised stem to half a pint of cold water macerated for three hours and strained; of this the dose is from one and a half to three ounces thrice daily; it is rendered more agreeable by the addition of Cinnamon, Cloves, or other aromatics. It has been used with benefit in mild forms of *Intermittent Fevers*, and in *Constitutional Debility, and Loss of Appetite after these and other Fevers.* It has also been found useful in some forms of *Dyspepsia*, and in *Chronic Rheumatism.*

353. An Extract (Sat-giló, *Hind. Punj.*; Gul-bél-kásat, *Duk.;* Sath-gilló'í, *Kash.*, Shíndal-sharuk-arai, *Tam.;* Palo, *Beng.;* Tippa-sattu, *Tel.*) prepared by the Native doctors, is held in high repute amongst them in *Intermittents, &c.* It is a white floury substance, with a strongly bitter taste. It is, however, often adulterated with, or consists altogether of, gluten of Wheat; its bitterness, therefore, is a good test of its quality. In doses of one to three drachms, it is highly esteemed as a tonic in *Debility after Fevers*, in *Spleen affections, &c.* Dr. Burton Brown speaks of it as an efficient remedy in *Diseases of the Bladder, especially in Chronic Inflammation of that organ.*

354. **Toddy.** A saccharine juice obtained by the excision of the spadix, or young flowering branch of the Palmyra, Cocoanut, and other Palms.

Séndí, Tárí (*Hind., Duk.*), Kallu (*Tam.*), Kallu (*Tel.*), Henda (*Can.*), Rá (*Cing.*), Tu-ak (*Malay*).

There are many kinds of Toddy in India, and they are named according to the plants from which they are produced. The names given above are generic.

355. Amongst its other uses Toddy is valuable as the basis of a very useful stimulant application, the TODDY POULTICE, which is to the Indian what the Yeast Poultice is to the European surgeon. It is prepared by adding freshly-drawn Toddy to Rice Flour till it has the consistence of a soft poultice, and subjecting the mixture in an open vessel to heat over a gentle fire, stirring constantly till fermentation commences, or it 'begins to rise,' as it is commonly expressed. This, spread on a cloth and applied to the parts, acts as a valuable stimulant application to *Gangrenous or Sloughing Ulcerations, Carbuncles, Indolent Ulcers, &c.* It hastens the separation of the slough and establishes subsequent healthy action.

356. Toddy left exposed to the air rapidly undergoes vinous fermentation, and becomes converted into ARRACK, one of the most intoxicating drinks of the country. This Arrack, subjected to distillation until it has a specific gravity of 0·920, may be employed as Proof Spirit in the preparation of tinctures and other pharmaceutical purposes, and in the formation of cold evaporating lotions (380).

357. **Turmeric.** The dried root-stock of Curcuma longa, *Linn.*

Halad, Haldí (*Hind., Duk., Punj.*), Holodí (*Beng.*), Lidar, Gandar-i-lidar, (*Kash.*), Manjal (*Tam.*), Pasupu (*Tel.*), Mannal, Marin-nala (*Mal.*),

Arishiná (*Can.*), Halede (*Mah.*), Halad (*Guz.*), Kahá (*Cing.*), Sanó, Tanún (*Burm.*), Kooneit (*Malay*).

358. Turmeric has been employed in the following affections with excellent effects :—

359. *In Catarrh, or severe 'Cold in the head,'* the fumes of burning Turmeric inhaled through the nostrils, act as a local stimulant or irritant, causing a considerable discharge of mucus from the nasal cavity ; this is generally followed by a marked degree of relief to the congestion or fulness often so troublesome in these cases.

360. *In Catarrhal and Purulent Ophthalmia*, especially in that termed '*Country Sore-Eye*,' a Decoction of Turmeric (one ounce of the bruised root to 20 ounces of water) proves a very effectual lotion for relieving the burning and moderating the urgency of the symptoms. A piece of soft rag soaked in it should be kept constantly over the affected eye.

361. **Oil of Turpentine.** The oil obtained by distillation from Pinus palustris, *Lamb.*, and other species of Pinus.

Gandhá-barójé-ká-tél (*Hind.*), Gandhá-férózé-ká-tél, Káfúr-ká-tailam (*Duk.*), Kapúrér-tail (*Beng.*), Karppúrat-tailam (*Tam.*), Karppúra-tailam (*Tel., Mal.*), Karapúrada-tailá (*Can.*), Kápúrácha-tela (*Mah.*), Karpúrnu-tél, Tarpintan (*Guz.*), Kapurutel (*Cing.*), Piyo-sí (*Burm.*), Nimiak Kapor Baroos (*Malay*).

362. Oil of Turpentine is procurable in most large bazaars, but not generally sufficiently pure for internal administration. It answers, however, perfectly well for external or local application, and is most valuable in the preparation of TURPENTINE STUPES or EPITHEMS, which are made in one of the following ways:—1. By steeping a flannel in hot water, as hot as can be borne by the hand, wringing it out dry and sprinkling the surface freely with Oil of Turpentine. 2. By steeping a piece of lint or rag of the required size in Oil of Turpentine, placing it over the affected surface, and immediately applying over it flannel heated before a fire, as hot as can be borne. In either way it acts admirably as a counter-irritant, and in most cases is superior to mustard poultices. It is applicable to all cases of *Internal Inflammations, Spasmodic Affections of the Bowels, advanced stages of Dysentery and Diarrhœa, Obstinate Vomiting, Flatulence, and Flatulent Colic, Chronic Bronchitis attended with Cough and Difficulty of Breathing, Asthma, &c.*

363. In some cases, greater benefit is derived from applying these Stupes to a distant point rather than near to the affected part; thus in *Apoplexy, Insensibility, Convulsions, Delirium,* whether arising in the course of fever or otherwise, they produce the best effects when applied to the feet and to the calves of the legs. *In Cholera,* when applied successively to the abdomen, over the region of the heart, along the spine and to the extremities, they often seem materially to aid other measures in stimulating the system and raising the vital powers. Turpentine friction

and turpentine enemas may also be resorted to as aids to other treatment.

363*b*. *In Pecnash*, or *Maggots in the Nose*, common amongst the natives of Bengal and other parts of India, 'the best treatment is to inject every opening in the skin of those affected with this disease with pure Oil of Turpentine, which is found to kill the maggots, and then to extract any maggots that are visible by means of a pair of forceps. Chloroform is even more efficacious, but is more expensive.' (Dr. T. E. B. Brown, *Indian Med. Gaz.*, Sept. 1879, p. 263.)

364. TURPENTINE ENEMAS (one ounce of the Oil to 15 ounces of Conjee) are valuable agents in many cases, as in *Apoplexy*, *Insensibility*, *Convulsions*, *especially in those after Childbirth*, *Hysterical Fits*, *Spasmodic Affections of the Bowels*, *Flatulence*, *Flatulent Colic*, *&c.* They, together with turpentine stupes, have sometimes excellent effects in stimulating the system and rousing the vital powers in *Delirium and Exhaustion attendant on Fever.*

365. *For the removal of Thread Worms from the Rectum and Lower Bowel*, a Turpentine Enema often proves effectual. In the treatment of *Tape Worm* Oil of Turpentine is a remedy of established value; it is best given internally in a dose of three drachms with an equal quantity of Castor Oil; the latter is considered to prevent the unpleasant head symptoms which are apt to arise when the Turpentine is given alone. It is best given two or three hours after a meal; if taken on an empty stomach it is apt to produce vomiting. The patient should remain quiet

after taking it, and broths and mucilaginous drinks should be taken to aid its operation. The Oil of Turpentine for this purpose should be obtained from a regular chemist or other reliable source.

366. TURPENTINE LINIMENT is a valuable application in *Chronic Rheumatism, Lumbago, Sciatica, and other forms of Neuralgia, in Chronic Enlargement of the Joints, Bruises, Sprains, Muscular Pains, &c.* It is formed by dissolving one ounce of Camphor in 16 ounces of Oil of Turpentine, and then adding two ounces of Soft Soap, rubbing them together until they are thoroughly mixed. *Chronic Coughs,* especially of the aged, are much benefited by this liniment well rubbed into the chest at night.

367. TURPENTINE OINTMENT is prepared by melting together at a gentle heat one ounce of Oil of Turpentine, 60 grains of White or Black Dammar (372), half an ounce of Yellow Wax, and half an ounce of Prepared Lard (or Kokum Butter). The ingredients, when melted together, should be removed from the fire, and the mixture constantly stirred whilst cooling. It constitutes a good stimulant application to *Indolent and ill-conditioned Ulcerations, &c.* Diluted with equal parts of lard (or ghee), it forms a highly useful dressing for *Carbuncles,* aiding the separation of sloughs, and stimulating to healthy action. It should be changed twice or thrice daily. Its action is aided by generous diet, &c., as mentioned in Index, Art. *Carbuncle.* Some *Chronic Skin Diseases* improve under the use of the undiluted ointment, but in those of the *Hairy Scalp of Parasitic origin,* the pure oil, locally

applied, according to Erlach (*Practitioner*, Oct. 1871), more surely and more rapidly than any other remedy.

367*b*. Tylophora, or Country Ipecacuanha. Tylophora asthmatica, *W. et A.*

Antá-múl, Janglí-pikván (*Hind.*), Pit-kárí (*Duk.*), Anto-mul (*Beng.*), Nach-churuppán, Náy-pálai, Péyp-pálai (*Tam.*), Verri-pála, Kukka-pála (*Tel.*), Valli-pála (*Mal.*), Bin-nuga (*Cing.*).

368. This plant is common in sandy localities in Bengal, and other parts of India. Its roots and leaves possess valuable emetic properties; the former, as met with in the bazaars, occurs in the form of thick, contorted pieces of a pale colour, and a bitterish, somewhat nauseous taste. As an emetic, and especially as a remedy in dysentery, it has long been in repute, but it has been superseded by the dried leaves, the operation of which has been found more uniform and certain; in fact, they are justly regarded as one of the best indigenous substitutes for Ipecacuanha. The dose of the powdered dried leaves as an emetic for an adult is from 40 to 50 grains; in smaller doses, four to eight grains, its action is that of an expectorant and diaphoretic.

369. *In Dysentery and Diarrhœa,* even in the earliest stages, and whilst fever is present, it may be given in doses of 10 to 15 grains three or four times daily, conjoined with mucilage; and Opium if required; or it may be commenced in one large dose in the same way as Ipecacuanha (see Index). If the dysentery be

connected with intermittent fever, or be of malarious origin, it should be combined with quinine.

370. *In Chronic Bronchitis, Coughs, Colds, and the early stage of Hooping Cough*, it has been administered with manifest benefit as an expectorant and diaphoretic, in doses of five grains thrice daily or oftener, either alone or combined with Syrup of Country Liquorice (6).

371. **Vateria Indica,** *Linn.*, **Resin of.** Piney, or White Dammar.*

Sufĕd-dámar (*Hind.*, *Duk.*), Kúndro (*Beng.*), Sundras (*Punj.*), Sindrus (*Kash.*), Vellai-kúndrikum (*Tam.*), Dúpa-dámaru, Tella-dámaru (*Tel.*), Vella-kúnturukkam (*Mal.*), Hal, Hal-dumlua (*Cing.*), Guttah rukam putch (*Malay*).

372. The specimens of White or Piney Dammar are met with in the bazaars in irregular masses, which differ in colour, fragrance, and density, some being of a light-greenish colour, dense and uniform in substance, whilst others are yellow amber-coloured, and vesicular, or full of small bladders; these differences apparently arise from the mode of collection and the age of the trees producing them. This resin burns with a clear steady light, giving off a pleasant smell, but very little smoke; under the influence of gentle heat it combines with wax and oil, and forms a good substitute

* In the absence of White Dammar, Black Dammar, the resin of Canarium strictum, *Roxb.* may be substituted. Its native names are Kalá-damar (*Hind.*, *Duk.*, *Beng.*), Karuppu-damar (*Tam.*), Nalla-rojan (*Tel.*), Kálo-damar (*Guz.*).

for officinal Resin in various ointments and plasters. The following is an eligible form for common use. Take of White Dammar, five ounces; Lard or Kokum Butter, eight ounces; Wax, two ounces. Melt with a gentle heat, stirring briskly as it cools. This spread on rag or lint forms a good stimulant dressing for *Carbuncles and other Ulcerations.*

373. From the fruit of Vateria Indica, *Linn.*, common on the western coast of the Peninsula, is obtained a solid fatty oil named PINEY TALLOW or VEGETABLE TALLOW OF CANARA, which has obtained considerable repute as a local application in *Chronic Rheumatism*, and some other painful affections. Like Kokum Butter, it may be used as a substitute for lard and other animal fats in the preparation of ointments, &c. It is deserving of more attention than has hitherto been paid to it.

373*a*. **Vernonia Seeds.** The seeds of Vernonia anthelmintica, *Willd.*

Sómráj, Bukchí (*Hind.*), Sómráj (*Beng.*), Káttu-shíragam (*Tam.*), Adavi-jila-kara, Visha-kanta-kálu (*Tel.*), Káttu-jírakam (*Mal.*), Kádu-jirage (*Can.*), Ránácha-jíré (*Mah.*), Kadvo-jíri (*Guz.*), Sanni-náegam, Sanni-násang (*Cing.*), Justan hutan (*Malay*).

373*b*. The plant which yields these seeds is common in waste places near villages throughout India, and the dried seeds are met with in almost every bazaar; they are about the eighth of an inch in length, of a dark brown colour, covered with whitish scattered hairs, cylindrical, tapering towards the base, marked with about ten paler longitudinal ridges, and crowned with a circle of short brown scales; taste, nauseous and bitter. These seeds enjoy a high repute amongst the natives as a vermifuge in cases of *Lumbrici or Round Worms*, which, under their use, are stated to be expelled in a lifeless state, thus showing that they exercise a specific influence on the worm. The ordinary dose of the bruised seed, administered in electuary with honey, is about two drachms, given in two equal doses at the interval of a few hours, and followed by an aperient. In this character they seem well worthy of further trials. In Travancore, the bruised seeds, ground up into a paste with lime-juice, are largely employed as a means of destroying *Lice* infesting the body. The reports received of their efficacy for this purpose justify further trials with them.

374. **Vinegar.**

Sirká (*Hind., Duk., Beng., Punj., Kash.*), Kádi (*Tam.*), Kádi-nóllu (*Tel.*), Káti (*Mal.*), Hulirasa (*Can.*), Kádi, Vená-kiri (*Cing.*), Pón-ye (*Burm.*), Chuka (*Malay*).

375. Many kinds of Vinegar are met with in India, but as they are of very varying strength and degree of purity, the imported English Distilled or White Wine Vinegar should be preferred, when procurable, as it generally may be in large bazaars, for medical purposes. In its absence, the best native kinds,

especially that prepared from the Toddy of the Palmyra tree, should be used.*

376. *In Smallpox, Measles, Scarlet Fever, and other Febrile Affections*, a mixture of one part of Vinegar and three of Water forms a soothing and refreshing application, with which the whole surface may be sponged twice or thrice daily, the temperature being regulated as described in Sect. 385. Sprinkled about the sick room, in these and other cases, undiluted vinegar acts in a degree as a deodorant, and is generally very agreeable to the patient.

377. *In Relaxed, Ulcerated, and other forms of Sore Throat, especially in that of Scarlet Fever, in Hoarseness*, &c., benefit is often derived from the inhalation of the vapour of hot Vinegar.

378. *In Phthisis*, sponging the chest with diluted Vinegar is said to be very effectual in allaying the *profuse perspirations.* A good mixture for this purpose is composed of one part of Vinegar, one of Eau de Cologne, and two of Water; it is a measure attended with salutary effects, and is generally of great comfort to the patient. *As a preventive of Phthisis* the practice has been strongly recommended of washing the chest every morning with Vinegar and Water, beginning with it tepid, and reducing the temperature gradually, until it can be used quite cold. The same measure persevered in has been found useful by persons

* At Pasham and on the frontier a very superior vinegar is manufactured from the juice of the grape; hence 'Pasham Vinegar' is well known throughout the Punjab and Kashmir, and even at Bombay and Kurrachee (*Dr. Aitchison*).

subject to repeated attacks of *Coughs and Asthmas;* it often seems to diminish the liability to a return of these attacks, and to act as a preventive.

379. *In Abortion and other forms of Uterine Hæmorrhage,* the continued application of cold Vinegar and Water to the pubes is not only agreeable to the patient, but tends considerably to arrest the discharge of blood. In the absence of better agents, Vinegar diluted and sweetened to taste may also be advantageously given internally. *Bleeding from the Nose* sometimes yields to a piece of rag saturated with Vinegar introduced into the nostril.

380. *To Bruises, Sprains, Contusions, and local Inflammations,* diluted Vinegar is a popular and useful application. An excellent 'EVAPORATING LOTION' in these cases is formed of equal parts of Vinegar, Arrack, and Water. This forms also a good application to the head in the *Headache and Delirium of Fever.* The pains of *Venomous Bites or Stings, e.g., of Scorpions, Centipedes, Wasps, Mosquitoes, &c.,* is often greatly relieved by the constant application of a piece of rag moistened with Vinegar.

381. *To Milk or Mammary Abscesses* warm Vinegar, perseveringly employed for twenty-four hours, is stated on good authority to be one of the best applications which can be used for relieving the congestion; it is particularly useful when the breasts are greatly and painfully distended with milk, and the earlier in the case it is employed, the greater are its chances of success.

382. *Particles of Lime (Chunam) in the Eye* are

effectually dissolved and the pain eased by bathing the eye with diluted Vinegar, not strong enough to cause smarting; it requires to be introduced between the eyelids.

383. **Water.**

Páni (*Hind.*, *Duk.*, *Beng.*, *Guz.*, *Mah.*, *Punj.*), Áb, Sag (*Kash.*), Ṭanni, Jalam, Nír (*Tam.*), Jalam, Níllu (*Tel.*), Vellam (*Mal.*), Vaturu (*Cing.*), Yé (*Burm.*), Ahyer (*Malay*).

384. Water for medicinal purposes, *e.g.*, making infusions, decoctions, &c., should be the purest which can be procured. At certain seasons, however, especially during the monsoon, the best water is apt to be so muddy as to be unfit either for medicinal or drinking use. Under these circumstances, recourse may be had to the native practice of rubbing the inside of a vessel or chattie with Clearing Nut,* bruised or sliced, previous to the water being poured into it. This simple measure is said to render the muddiest water clear and wholesome. Where water has been collected from swampy or malarious localities, a better plan is to subject it (with the addition of a piece of freshly prepared charcoal) to *boiling*, and subsequent straining or filtering. The uses of water in medicine are multifarious and important.

* The Seeds of Strychnos Potatorum, *Linn.*. Nir-malí (*Hind.*, *Beng.*, *Mah.*, and *Guz.*), Chil-bínj (*Duk.*), Tétrán-kottai (*Tam.* and *Malyal.*), Tétrán-parala (*Tel.*), Ingini-atta (*Cing.*), Kamou-yeki (*Burm.*).

385. *As a drink in Fever and Inflammations*, cold water may be taken without restriction, and it may be rendered more refrigerant and agreeable by the addition of some mucilaginous agents, as rice, &c., and some vegetable acid, as tamarind pulp or lime-juice. For *Irritability of Stomach and Vomiting in Fever*, water drunk as hot as it can be borne will often prove very effectual; 'But,' observes Dr. Aitchison, 'the remedy should not consist of merely a mouthful or so of hot water; but of two or three tumblers full. One would suppose that drinking this amount of water on an irritable stomach, would rather produce vomiting: this is not the case. The patient may bring up a little of the water; but usually he simply turns round, and falls asleep as if a narcotic had been given him.' *In Smallpox, Measles, Scarlatina, and other Fevers*, the practice of freely sponging the surface once or twice daily with water is extremely grateful and refreshing to the patient, and may be used with perfect safety unless the heat be high above the natural standard, when tepid water should be substituted. As a general rule, the temperature of the water should be regulated by the patient's feelings; it should be cold, tepid, or quite warm, as is most agreeable. A mixture of Vinegar and Water (one part of the former to three of the latter) is even more refreshing than plain water.

386. *In Sunstroke*, the first thing to be done after removing the patient into the shade and taking off the head-gear and upper clothing, is to practise COLD

AFFUSION. For this purpose he should be held in a sitting posture, whilst the water, the colder the better, is poured down in a pretty full stream, at a height of two or three feet over the head, spine, and chest. After its application for a minute or two, the patient will probably heave a deep sigh or inspiration, when the affusion should be discontinued and the patient removed to a dry spot, thoroughly dried with a warm cloth or towel, and diligent friction maintained till full consciousness is restored. Mustard poultices (247), Turpentine stupes (362) to the feet and calves are also advisable if insensibility be long continued. One or two points demand attention. 1. The water should not descend all at once, but rather in a small continuous stream, and it should be directed not so much on the top of the head as on the back part and upper portion of the spine. 2. It should at once be discontinued when the patient begins to revive. 3. It is not adapted for the aged and debilitated, or when the skin is cold and clammy; in these cases affusion should be restricted to dashing cold water on the face and chest, together with persevering frictions of the extremities; and when the patient is able to swallow, administering mild stimulants, *e.g.*, ammonia, weak brandy and water, &c. The above treatment is adapted for *Apoplexy and Profound Insensibility, such as occurs in Poisoning by Opium, Bish (Aconite), or the fumes of Datura.* In ordinary cases of *Fainting, Convulsions in Adults arising from no evident cause, and Hysterical Convulsions in Women,* simply dashing cold water with some little degree of violence on the face and bosom, is generally all that is required.

387. *In the Convulsions of Infancy and Childhood,* the little patient should be put into a hot bath, with as little delay as possible, the head at the same time being slightly elevated, and enveloped in cloths kept wet with cold water, the colder the better. Under the simultaneous use of the hot bath and the cold lotion to the head, aided by the exhibition of a dose of Castor Oil, the convulsions will often speedily subside. The bath should be as hot as can be borne, about 98° F., and the child should remain in it for ten or fifteen minutes, but the cold to the head may be continued for some hours. Should the convulsions return, the bath may be repeated, followed by small Mustard poultices (247) applied to the feet. A hot bath is also very useful in allaying *Colic in Children.*

388. *To check violent Hæmorrhage or Flooding after Labours,* nothing is much more effectual than dashing *cold* water in a pretty full stream, and with some little degree of force, over the abdominal surface, especially the lower portion. At the same time, a piece of soft rag, made into a pyramidical form, thoroughly saturated with cold water, or vinegar and water (in equal parts), should be introduced into the vagina. After the flooding has been subdued, the external application of cold water, or vinegar and water, should be kept on for some time. *N.B.* —During a confinement in India, it should be an invariable rule, to meet such an emergency as the above, to have ready at hand two or three chatties

of *cold* water, for a patient may die from loss of blood if the water has to be fetched from a distant source.

389. *In Cholera*, the free use of cold water as a drink appears materially to aid other treatment, of whatsoever kind that may be; it should be as cold as procurable, iced if possible, and taken in large and repeated draughts; although the first four or five draughts may be rejected, its use should still be persevered in; the stomach will eventually retain it, and when this is effected, a beneficial change in the state of the patient generally takes place. Whatever other treatment is adopted, cold water (iced if possible) in copious draughts is a valuable auxiliary, perfectly safe, agreeable to the patient, and likely to be productive of the best effects.

390. *Many forms of Sore Throat, and Coughs attended with Difficulty of Breathing and Scanty Expectoration*, are much benefited by repeated inhalations of hot water, and their efficiency is increased by the addition of mucilaginous agents, as Abelmoschus (1). *In Croup*, relays of sponges filled with water, as hot as the little patient can bear, should be applied immediately beneath the chin, along the whole course of the throat. They should be persevered in for half an hour, and then discontinued if they fail to produce benefit. In severe cases, Turpentine stupes (362) prove more serviceable.

392. *In many painful affections of the Kidneys, Bladder, and Uterus, in the passage of Gall Stones*, and in *Retention of the Urine from Spasmodic Stricture consequent on a debauch or exposure*, the hot hip-bath proves highly serviceable and soothing.

393. Hot-water Fomentations are very serviceable in many cases, *e.g.*, *Local Inflammations, Incipient Abscesses, Boils, Sprains, Lumbago, Colic and Spasmodic Affections of the Bowels, Congestion of the Liver, Asthma, &c.* To obtain their full effect, a few points require to be attended to. 1. The water should be as hot as can be borne. 2. Two or more thickly folded cloths (if flannel so much the better) of a size rather larger than the surface they are to cover, should be in readiness. 3. One of these having been removed from the water, should be thoroughly wrung, so that it should hold no superfluous moisture, and should be immediately applied to the surface. 4. A second cloth having been got ready in the same way, the first, after the lapse of two or three minutes, should be removed, and the second applied. This process should be continued for half an hour if necessary, care being taken that the water be kept at the original temperature by means of fresh relays, and that there should be no longer interval than possible between the removal of one and the application of the succeeding fomentation. Subsequently, care should be taken to protect the fomented part from exposure to cold draughts of air. Some forms of *severe Headache, especially those occurring in Fevers*, are far more benefited by hot-water fomentations, or stupes thus applied, than from cold lotions commonly employed for the purpose. According to Dr. Aitchison, nothing relieves the *Headache or great fulness of the Head in Fevers* so effectually as the continuous application of extremely hot-water stupes to the nape of the neck. *The Irritative Bilious Diarrhœa*

of these Fevers, he adds, is more frequently improved and arrested by large warm-water enemas, administered at least morning and evening, than by any other remedy he knows of.

394. *In the treatment of Wounds, Ulcers, and Inflamed Surfaces*, 'WATER DRESSING' possesses many advantages, especially in tropical regions, over poultices and ointments. The process is exceedingly simple, consisting only of a piece of lint of thick texture, and of a size sufficient completely to cover the wound, soaked in tepid water. This is placed on the affected part, and the whole enveloped in an ample piece of oiled silk, so as effectually to prevent evaporation. Young plantain leaf answers the purpose as well as oiled silk. Cold water may be substituted for tepid, should it be more agreeable to the feelings of the patient.

395. *Sloughing and Gangrenous Ulcerations, and Carbuncles ('Rajah Boils') after suppuration*, are more effectually treated by what is termed 'IRRIGATION,' which consists in keeping up a continuous stream of water, tepid or cold, as the patient may prefer, for half an hour twice daily. A common kettle, or one of the Natives' drinking-vessels provided with a spout, answers well for the purpose, and it should be held so that the fall of water should be about a foot, or rather more, but the height should be regulated in a measure by the patient's feelings. If pain is caused, the height should be diminished. With each irrigation, more or less of the slough comes away, and in a few days the ulcer will, in most instances, assume a healthy

appearance, when it may be treated as an ordinary ulcer—with cold water dressing, Turpentine, or Wax Ointment, &c. In the intervals between the irrigations, Toddy Poultices (355) should be applied.

396. Another way in which Water may be utilized is in the formation of a VAPOUR BATH, which is often a most serviceable resource in *Chronic Rheumatism, Obstinate Skin Diseases, Dropsical Affections, the early stages of Diabetes, and in all cases where the skin is dry, rough, and not much above the natural standard.* It is inadvisable in fever cases. *Incipient Colds and Catarrhs* following exposure to wet, &c., may often be speedily arrested by a vapour bath, taken immediately before going to bed at night.

397. The Vapour Bath apparatus, which should be kept ready in all large establishments in India, consists of a bamboo frame of a conical shape, covered with wax-cloth or some other impervious material; it should be large enough to enclose the whole body (when the patient is in a sitting posture), and an aperture with a loose frill attached, so as to tie round the patient's throat, should be left at the apex. Under this the patient, divested of his clothing, should sit with the head and face projecting through the opening at the top, and a chattie, or open vessel, of boiling water having been introduced, sweating soon commences and should be kept up for a quarter of an hour or more. Then the patient should be thoroughly dried with warm, rough towels and go to bed, or to some other place where he will be effectually protected from draughts of cold air.

397*b*. THE WET SHEET has been highly spoken of in the treatment of *Delirium Tremens;* it is applied as follows :—Strip the patient naked and roll him in a wet sheet till he looks like a mummy, and then roll a blanket round this again. In many cases the delirious excitement will subside as soon as a hot vapour surrounds the patient, and he will fall into a quiet sleep. It should be used with caution in the case of an old debilitated drunkard.

398. **Wax.**

Móm (*Hind.*, *Duk.*, *Beng.*, *Punj.*), Si'úth (*Kash.*), Mozhukka (*Tam.*), Máinam (*Tel.*), Mezhuka (*Mal.*), Ména (*Can.*, *Mah.*), Mín (*Guz.*), Ittí (*Cing.*), Phayoui (*Burm.*), Libu lubah (*Malay*).

399. Wax, obtainable of good quality in most bazaars, has no especial medicinal properties; it is, however, extensively used in the formation of ointments, plasters, &c., for the purpose of giving them consistence, and a mildly stimulant action. The following is stated to be an excellent stimulant application to '*Blind Boils,*' so common at certain seasons in many parts of India; it is thought to bring them to a head sooner than any other remedy. Take of Indian Bdellium,* Wax, and Sesamum oil, of each one ounce; melt together with a gentle heat, stirring well, and strain. A portion of this, spread on rag or lint, should be placed over each boil. It is also a good dressing for subsequent *Ulceration.*

* Gúgul (*Hind.*, *Punj.*), Kánt-i-gun (*Kash.*), the gum resin of Balsamodendron Mukul (*Hooker*), and B. pubescens (*Stocks*).

ADDENDA.

400. **Cinchona Febrifuge, or Darjeeling Cinchona Alkaloid.**

In 1875 Mr. Wood, the Government Quinologist, prepared from the bark of Cinchona succirubra and other species under cultivation at Darjeeling an alkaloid, or rather a mixture of alkaloids, which has received the provisional names of 'DARJEELING CINCHONA ALKALOID,' and 'CINCHONA FEBRIFUGE.' A rough analysis shows that it contains—Quinine, 15·5; Cinchonidine, 29·0; Cinchonine, 33·5; Amorphous Alkaloid, 17·0; and Colouring Matter, 5·0 in 100 parts. It occurs in the form of a buff-coloured powder, of a peculiar disagreeable smell, and bitter, nauseous taste; insoluble in water, soluble in mineral and vegetable acids.

401. In the treatment of *Intermittent Fever* this remedy ranks next to Quinine, over which it possesses the advantage of being comparatively cheap, and, from its being manufactured in India, is within the reach of all. It has its disadvantages, however, being apt to create nausea, vomiting, with a burning sensation at the pit of the stomach, extending, in some instances, to the throat, and occasionally diarrhœa. Like Quinine, if given in sufficient doses to produce its

specific effect, it gives rise to headache, singing in the ears, giddiness, and other symptoms included under the term 'Quinism;' but all these pass away on the discontinuance of the remedy, leaving no after ill effects. It is, in fact, a thoroughly safe and efficacious remedy in ordinary simple Intermittents, but its use is limited to these. In the severer forms and in Remittent Fevers it is not to be depended upon: here Quinine remains the sheet anchor. The dose is from five to ten grains twice or thrice daily during the intermission or in anticipation of an expected paroxysm. Dilute Sulphuric Acid (one and a half minim to one grain of the alkaloid) is said to be the best solvent, but given with Dilute Hydrochloric or Citric Acid, its disagreeable taste and smell are partially masked, and hence is more easily borne. Fresh Lime Juice is recommended as an eligible vehicle for popular use.

402. *In Debility after Fevers* it promises to be of great value as a tonic, given in small doses. It is worthy of a trial in *Enlargement of the Spleen* in combination with Sulphate of Iron (176). In *Neuralgia, Face Ache, Tic Doloureux,* when assuming a periodical form, this remedy is well worthy of a fair trial. It should be given in full doses (ten grains) thrice daily for adults.

403. Closely allied to the foregoing is another form of collective Cinchona Alkaloids, to which its discoverer, Dr. de Vrij, has given the name of QUINETUM. It is said to represent the whole of the alkaloids in Cinchona succirubra bark in proportion of Quinine, 25; Cinchonidine, 50; and Cinchonine, 20 in 100 parts. Dr. Vinkhuysen, who tried it extensively in

the treatment of *Intermittent Fevers*, says that 'Quinetum is of great value as a febrifuge, but that it takes longer to act, and will not replace Quinine in pernicious fever. It has the same apyretic effect as Quinine, but is less powerful; larger doses are therefore required at longer intervals before the paroxysms. It produces no ill effects, no noises in the ear, and can be taken by those who cannot take Quinine. It is more efficacious in chronic cases and as a tonic, whilst in masked malaria it is incomparably superior to Quinine.' This statement is quoted from Sir Joseph Fayrer's valuable work 'On the Climate and Fevers of India' (London, 1882), and to it he (Sir Joseph) adds the expression of his own belief that 'it is a very valuable drug.' We learn from the same authority that it is now largely prepared in India. This being the case, and as it is less than half the price of Quinine, it may be regarded as an important addition to Indian Materia Medica. The dose is from eight to sixteen grains in diluted Lime Juice or other acidulated water.

404. **Kerosine Oil.**

Pathar-ka-tél (*Punj.*).

405. Owing to the extensive use of this mineral Oil for lighting purposes during the past few years, it can now be obtained in nearly every bazaar in the country. According to the experience of Dr. Aitchison, no local remedy is so pre-eminently useful in all *Skin Diseases* as this, especially when of a parasitic origin. It is comparatively of little use in syphilitic eruptions.

The oil may be employed pure when no large surface is involved, but if the disease to be treated extensively covers the body, it should be diluted with equal parts of sweet oil. Nothing can come up to it, he asserts, in removing and *destroying bugs* from old wood. It is also said to be of use in *removing white ants.*

406. *In Itch*, when of limited extent, after opening each pustule, rub into the part carefully twice or thrice daily pure Kerosine Oil. If it be extensively diffused over the whole body, after thoroughly washing with soap and water, rub in a solution of equal parts of Kerosine and Sweet Oil. This, observes Dr. Aitchison, far surpasses the Sulphur treatment. *In Ringworm* it is sufficient to paint the affected spot with the pure oil twice or thrice daily. *In Scald Head*, after cutting the hair as short as possible, apply a poultice to clean off the scab from the scalp, and then thoroughly saturate the cleansed surface with Kerosine Oil. During treatment the patient should wear an oil-skin cap. Oil alone, applied thus, adds Dr. A., will cure the disease, but Kerosine does it more quickly and effectually. *Lice* of all kinds are at once destroyed by rubbing Kerosine Oil into the parts they occupy, and are totally exterminated by two or three free applications. (Dr. Atchison.)

407. **Sugar.**

Shakar (*Hind., Duk.*), Bhúra, Chiní (*Beng.*), Misri (*Punj.*), Sakkará, Sharukkarai (*Tam.*), Shakkara (*Tel.*), Sharkkara, Panjasára (*Mal.*), Síní, Sakkere (*Cing.*), Saghia or Tagiya (*Burm.*), Gúla (*Mal.*).

408. This article is not usually regarded as a medicine, but Dr. Aitchison in his valuable notes, points out how he has utilized it as such with excellent effect; and as it is procurable throughout the length and breadth of India, it seems well worthy of notice in this place. Only the best and purest kinds should be employed for medicinal purposes.

409. In all forms of *Ophthalmia* (*Country Sore Eyes, &c.*), Dr. A. states that he has found a solution of one drachm of Sugar in three drachms of Water dropped into the eye every hour or so, never fail to afford relief, and that generally, if applied early, cuts short the disease at once. This practice, he adds, he has followed for twelve years, and used nothing else. Children, according to his experience, will actually come and ask to have the remedy dropped into their eyes, so great is the relief it affords. At bedtime, in these cases, it is advisable to apply to the eyelashes a little sweet oil or grease, and the first thing in the morning carefully to wash the eyes with hot milk and water. This solution is also useful for *removing small foreign substances from the Eye.*

410. *In Gonorrhœa and Vaginal Discharges* the above solution is an excellent application, though not so uniformly useful as in Ophthalmia. In Gonorrhœa, it may be commenced with at once, the injections being repeated frequently during the day, in addition to general remedies; but in Vaginal discharges other remedies may be tried first. (See Index.)

411. Sugar is an excellent dressing for certain forms of *Foul, Gangrenous looking Ulcers,* the Sugar (white or refined) in grain being merely sprinkled over the sore which under its use soon assumes a healthy appearance. As a drawing plaster for *Boils,* equal parts of Sugar and Yellow Soap, is an old remedy. (Dr. Aitchison.)

412. **Petroleum. Rock Oil.**

Mittí-ká-têl (*Hind., Duk.*), Mátiyá-tail (*Beng.*), Man-yenney, Man-tayilam (*Tam., Mal.*), Manti-tayilam, Manti-núné (*Tel.*), Mannunyanné (*Can.*), Mattí-cha-téla (*Mah.*), Mattí-nu-tel (*Guz.*), Yé-ná (*Burm.*).

413. Petroleum, a mineral oil, semi-liquid somewhat of the consistence of treacle, tenacious, semi-transparent of a deep sherry red or nearly opaque, tar-like brown, with a peculiar though not unpleasant aromatic odour and pungent acrid taste, exudes spontaneously from the rocks in volcanic regions, and collects on the surface of certain lakes in Persia, Burmah, Assam, and the islands on the Arracan Coast, as well as in Barbadoes, Trinidad, and other West Indian Islands. As a medicinal agent, it is a terebinthinate (turpentine-like) stimulant, and as such appears to act specially on the kidneys, increasing in a marked degree the urinary secretion. The dose is about half a fluid drachm (thirty drops) suspended in mucilage.

414. Petroleum is very generally employed by

the Native practitioners externally as a stimulant in *Paralytic Affections* and in *Chronic Rheumatism,* and Dr. Fleming (Cat. p. 53), commenting on this, adds that he can, from his own experience, recommend it in the latter disease as an efficacious remedy, having derived more benefit from it than from the more costly Cajeput Oil, which he had previously used. A case of *Beri-beri* successfully treated by it, externally and internally, is recorded by Mr. S. Arokeum (*Madras Quart. Med. Journ.*, July 1863), but how far the recovery was due in this instance to the Petroleum seems doubtful. Still it seems worthy of further trials in this obscure affection.

415. *In Skin Diseases,* it is a useful external application, and a case of *Chronic Eczema,* which had resisted a host of remedies cured by it, is recorded by Dr. J. W. Mudge (*Indian Ann. of Med. Science,* 1854, p. 450). He used it incorporated with Soap in the proportion of a drachm to an ounce.

416. *As an Antiseptic agent in Surgical Practice,* some trials have been made with it by Sir Joseph Fayrer (*Indian Med. Gazette,* Sept. 1869, p. 184), and he comes to the conclusion that it possesses some if not all the advantages assigned to Carbolic Acid in this character. He used it, pure or diluted, with equal parts of oil or glycerine; and he states that whilst it certainly has some deodorising power, it appeared also to have that of limiting suppuration and of restraining the development of septic miasmata in the discharges. He likewise found it useful as a stimulating and detergent application to *Sloughing and Ulcerated*

Surfaces, and in one case of *Carbuncle* it proved most efficacious. It causes little inconvenience beyond slight smarting. 'The evidence of its virtue,' Sir J. Fayrer observes, 'is as yet but limited, yet it is such as to suggest the advantage of making further trial of what may prove to be a valuable addition to our surgical resources, and it has the advantage of being produced in the country.' The summaries of twenty cases are appended to illustrate the use of this hydrocarbon. It is to be hoped it will meet with further trials.

417. **Rock Salt**, an impure Chloride of Sodium.

Senda-lon, Senda-namak (*Hind.*, *Duk.*), Indúppú (*Tam.*, *Tel.*), Intúppa (*Mal.*).

418. Rock Salt occurs in large masses varying in weight from 2 or 3 to 8 or 10 lbs.; dull or brownish-white externally, white and crystalline internally, of a pure saline taste; procurable in all large Indian bazaars at four or five annas per lb. Though known to be a mere variety of Chloride of Sodium (common salt) it is possessed of far stronger purgative properties, it is also stronger than Cream of Tartar; but like this, it is not a satisfactory cathartic given alone; in combination with other purgatives, however, it is equal if not superior to it, and may advantageously replace it in Kaladana and other officinal Powders. (Dr. Moodeen Sheriff.)

COOKERY FOR THE SICK.

419. Mutton Broth and Beef Tea.

Take a pound of meat, free from fat; chop it up fine, and let it stand for one hour in a pint of cold water. Then add half a dozen Okra (1) cut transversely, and boil at a gentle heat to half a pint; strain and flavour with salt and pepper to taste. It should be freshly prepared daily.

420. Chicken Broth.

This is prepared in the same manner as the preceding, a full-grown fowl being substituted for the pound of meat. The two essential points to be attended to being, that the flesh is cut small or well bruised, and that it stands for an hour in cold water previous to being put on the fire. Half-grown fowls will answer for children. Like the preceding, it should be prepared fresh daily.

421. Raw Meat Juice.

The juice of raw meat is an invaluable remedy in sickness, more especially in the many diseases of the intestinal canal from which Europeans suffer in India, whether during infancy or in adult life. For obtaining this juice any meat will do, but beef is to be preferred. From a piece, say, a pound in weight, remove all the fat; then mince the meat; after which cover the mince with as much water as it will absorb in four or five minutes; then reduce the soft mass into a pulp in a mortar by means of a pestle. Pass this pulp through a cloth forcibly: the fluid which passes through the cloth is meat juice. Children will take this readily without any addition being made to it. Adults, however, frequently cannot do so, owing to its peculiar raw odour. In such cases it can be made palatable by the addition of a little salt, sometimes sherry, Worcester sauce, or even a little acid jelly; but whatever is done to this juice to make it palatable, on no account add mineral acids, or cook it, as in both cases the albumen of the juice becomes coagulated, making it less digestible. Where ice is procurable, meat in this form can be conveniently kept fresh for more than forty eight hours. Where ice cannot be obtained, and the climate is at summer heat, the juice should be extracted from the meat fresh each time it is to be given. (Dr. Aitchison.)

422. Rice Milk.

Boil one table spoonful of ground Rice with a pint and a half of Milk, or equal parts of milk and water; stir it smooth, and boil for two minutes; flavour with sugar and nutmeg. A very nourishing food for children.

423. Arrowroot.

Take a table spoonful of the best Arrowroot, and make it into a thin paste with a little water; then add gradually half a pint of boiling water, stirring it the whole time. Put it on the fire for two or three minutes, still continuing to stir it till the whole is uniformly mixed; then remove it from the fire and add grated nutmeg, sugar, &c., to taste. If made with milk instead of water, it is more nourishing, but when the stomach is weak it sometimes disagrees, and then water is preferable. It should be prepared fresh when required.

424. Sago.

Add a table spoonful of the best Sago to a pint of Water, and let it stand for two hours, then boil for a quarter of an hour, stirring the whole time, till it forms a clear uniform jelly. Remove from the fire, and flavour with sugar, nutmeg, &c.

425. Pish-Pash (Puss-Pass).

This is a regular Indian dish for invalids, and consists of fresh meat cooked amongst rice. Usually a chicken is cut up into small pieces, put into the bottom of a small pan, to which are added three table spoonfuls of rice, well cleaned, and over the whole is poured two breakfast cups full of cold water. This is now allowed to cook over a slow fire for three or four hours. Spices and salt, of course, can be added during the cooking process. If the patient is extremely ill the rice part alone is used, which has absorbed nearly the whole of the strength of the meat. Besides being given to invalids, this is a common diet amongst European children in India. (Dr. Aitchison.)

426. **Brandy Mixture.**

Take of Brandy and of Water each four table spoonfuls, the yolks of two Eggs, and half an ounce of powdered white Sugar. Beat the yolks and sugar well together, then add the spirit and water, and flavour with grated cinnamon or nutmeg.

This is a valuable stimulant and restorative in the low forms and advanced stages of *Fever*, *Smallpox*, *Measles*, *Exhausting Hæmorrhages*, *Cholera*, and other cases where the vital powers are greatly depressed. The dose for adults is from one to three table spoonfuls repeated according to circumstances; for children from a tea spoonful to a table spoonful according to age or the urgency of the symptoms.

427. *In Delirium Tremens* this is one of the best forms of stimulant, combining as it does nutritive with stimulant properties; indeed, when other food is rejected, the proportion of eggs may be doubled or trebled. In the young and vigorous, and in first attacks, all alcoholic drinks may be safely and strictly withheld, but should there be a great craving for drink, Omum Water (320) may be tried, as it is said to relieve this condition. In the old debilitated confirmed drinker, however, stimulants become a necessity, and Brandy Mixture in doses of one to two ounces may be given at stated intervals as required, but the patient should not be allowed to sip it, or take it occasionally as he thinks fit.

428. **White Wine Whey.**

Take one pint of fresh Milk, add Mace, Nutmeg

and Cinnamon, with Sugar to taste. Put it on a clear slow fire, stirring until the milk is on the point of boiling over. Then take it off, and throw in one or two wine glassfuls of Sherry or Madeira. Put it on the fire again, stirring it gently one way until it curdles; then remove, and strain through cloth or muslin. This taken at bedtime, the patient being well covered with clothes, so as to produce copious perspiration, has often an excellent effect in arresting incipient attacks of *Catarrh, Influenza, &c.*

429. **Egg Wine.**

Beat up one Egg (both yolk and white) with a table spoonful of cold Water. On this pour a mixture of a glass of Sherry and half a glass of water previously heated together (not boiling), stirring all the time. Then sweeten with white sugar, and add a little grated nutmeg, to taste. Taken in this form it is more digestible, but its flavour is improved by heating the ingredients in a clean saucepan over a gentle fire (not to boiling), stirring them one way till they thicken. This, with a small piece of toast or biscuit, may be advantageously taken by invalids twice daily, or as occasion requires.

430. **Strengthening Jelly.**

Steep two ounces of Isinglass or Prepared Gelatine, one ounce of Gum Arabic, five ounces of Sugar Candy, and a grated Nutmeg in a bottle of Port wine all night. In the morning, simmer over a slow fire till quite dissolved; then strain and set aside in a cool place till it forms a firm jelly. A piece the size of a nutmeg may be taken five or six times a day. This jelly is admirably suited for cases of debility when the stomach is unable to bear animal food.

PART II.

SYNOPSIS OR INDEX OF DISEASES.

The numbers have reference to the paragraphs; the asterisk (*) denotes those most deserving of attention.

Abdomen, Flatulent Distention of. See *Flatulence.*

Abortion. Use Vinegar externally and internally (379); if great restlessness or pain is present, give Opium (289); if the hæmorrhage continue unabated, apparently from want of power in the uterus to contract, try Borax and Cinnamon (58), or administer a Turpentine enema (364).† With these exceptions, let nature complete her work by herself; more harm than good may result from meddlesome interference. Perfect rest of mind and body, a strictly recumbent posture in a cool, well-ventilated apartment, and careful avoidance of all stimulant articles of diet and mental excitement, are essentials to successful treatment. *Threatened Abortion from a fall, over-exertion, &c.,* may sometimes be averted by a dose of Opium (289), and strict attention to the above hygienic rules. See also *Hæmorrhage, Internal.*

† In cases where there is much hæmorrhage, which does not abate under the above means, the Acetate of Lead and Opium Pills advised for *Hæmorrhage Internal* (foot-note), may be given with signal advantage.

Abscess. In the early stage apply Hot Water Fomentations (393); if there be much inflammation and pain, apply Leeches (215), and keep constantly to the part a solution of Sal Ammoniac (325), or Evaporating Lotion (380). If matter forms, apply Rice Poultices (322); when it comes so near the surface that it can be felt fluctuating under the finger, the abscess should be opened with a lancet at the most prominent point; and after the matter has been evacuated by gentle pressure, the Rice Poultices should be continued, and changed twice or thrice daily. Should the pain be so great as to prevent sleep, a dose of Opium (283) or Tincture of Datura (128) at bed-time is advisable. Should the discharge be profuse, and the patient weak, support the strength with a liberal diet and tonics, as Chiretta (98, 99), or Country Sarsaparilla (163), or Ním Bark (260). N.B.—Abscesses in the neck should only be opened by a doctor, or by one who is conversant with the anatomy of the part.

Acidity of the Stomach. See *Stomach, Acidity of.*

Acids, Poisoning with. Give copious draughts of Lime Water (228) and milk, or, if this be not at hand, soap and water, or chalk, or the plaster of the apartment beaten up with water. Rice Conjee (322) and other mucilaginous drinks, white of eggs, or draughts containing any bland oil, should be given freely. Much of the success in these cases depends upon the promptitude with which the remedies are applied.

Ague. See *Fever, Intermittent.*

Ague Cake. See *Spleen, Enlargement of.*

Apoplexy. If the patient is young and vigorous, pour cold water from a height on the head and spine as directed in 386. Keep Evaporating Lotion (380) to the head; give a Croton Pill (120), or if the patient is unable to swallow, place a drop or two of Croton Oil (121) at the back of the tongue. Apply Turpentine Stupes (363) or Mustard Poultices to the feet and calves. Should the insensibility continue, give a Turpentine enema (364). For the old and debilitated, and for natives generally, a little Brandy Mixture (426), or other stimulant judiciously given, offers a better prospect of success than bloodletting, which should never be had recourse to except under medical supervision.

Appetite, Loss of. First try Chiretta (98, 99*); should this fail, give one of the following: Sweet Flag Root (12), Country Sarsaparilla (163), Ním Bark (260), or Gulancha (352). Stomachics, as Capsicum (79), Cinnamon (102), or Cloves (105), may be advantageously combined with them, care being taken at the same time to regulate the bowels.

Arsenic, Poisoning with. As speedily as possible empty the stomach by an emetic of Sulphate of Copper (117) or Mustard (246), and then give copious draughts of white of eggs beaten up in milk, or a mixture of equal parts of Lime Water and Sesamum, Cocoa-nut, or other bland Oil. Powdered Sugar has been advised in these cases, but if of any service, it can only act like the preceding mixtures, mechanically, by enveloping the particles of the poison; this remark applies also to Powdered Charcoal, which has also been well spoken of. When the vomiting has abated, give a full dose of Castor Oil (84) to carry off any of the poison which may have passed into the intestines, and this may be repeated every day for two or three days. Should there be great exhaustion, a little stimulant, as Brandy Mixture (426), may be given, and a dose of Opium may be advisable, to subdue any subsequent great pain and restlessness.

Asthma. To relieve the severity of a paroxysm, try one or more of the following: Turpentine Stupes (362*), or Hot Water Fomentations to the chest (393), Camphor (70*), or Assafœtida (37) internally, and the inhalation of the fumes of Nitre Paper (268*) or of Datura (129*). A cup of hot, strong, milkless, sugarless Coffee, 'café noir,' drunk as hot as can be borne, sometimes gives great relief. Daily sponging the chest with Vinegar is thought to act in a measure as a preventive (378). A better preventive is the careful regulation of diet. Many a fit of asthma can be clearly traced to a hot supper, or some other error of diet.

Atrophy, or Wasting of the Body. Try Fish Liver Oil (142), with tonics, as Chiretta (98, 99), and change of air.

Bed Sores. To prevent these, bathe the parts daily with a solution of Camphor in spirit (75), or with Brandy or Eau de Cologne, or apply Alum and White of Egg (31*), and relieve the local pressure as much as possible by change of position, &c. A small circular pillow with a hollow centre (just like the pads worn by the Coolies on their heads in carrying weights, only thinner) is most useful for this purpose. Should a sore form notwithstanding, it should be treated as an ordinary ulcer. See *Ulcer.*

Beri-beri, Petroleum (414).

Bish (Aconite Root), Poisoning with. Strong stimulants, as Brandy and Ammonia; Cold Water Affusion (386), and persistent friction of the limbs and spine, appear to offer the best chance of success. Decoction of Galls (152) has been advised as an antidote. Strong hot Coffee (café noir) is worth a trial, if the patient can swallow.

Bites, Venomous, and Stings, e.g., of Centipedes, Scorpions, Wasps. All that is required in ordinary or mild cases, after immediate suction of the bite, is application of Vinegar (380), or Alum (32), or a strong solution of salt and water. Inunction of warm oil has been highly recommended. If Ipecacuanha is at hand, a small portion of it made into a thick paste with a few drops of water, and locally applied, is said in many instances to afford great and immediate relief. Brown Sugar is said to be specially useful in *Wasp Stings.* Soda is also said speedily to relieve the pain in these cases. Should the symptoms be severe, as is sometimes the case, Liquor Ammoniæ and stimulants, as advised for Snake Bites (Appendix B), should be given.

Bladder, Painful Affections and Irritable States of, are best relieved by Opium (286*), the free use of demulcents, as the Decoctions of Abelmoschus (2), Ispaghúl seeds (305), or Rice Conjee (322), and the use of the Hip Bath (392). The Extract of Gulancha (353) seems well worthy of a trial, especially in *Chronic Inflammation of the Bladder.*

Bleeding. See *Hæmorrhage.*

Blows. See *Sprains.*

Boils are to be treated much in the same way as Abscesses, by Hot Water Fomentations (393), Sal Ammoniac Lotion (332), and Rice Poultices (322). Leeches (212) are rarely necessary, unless there should be much pain and inflammation. Decoction of Country Sarsaparilla (163) may be given internally if there is any constitutional disturbance. A popular and useful 'drawing plaster' is a compound of equal weights of Brown Sugar and English Yellow Soap; a still better one is the ointment described in paragraph 399; a portion of either of these spread on rag should be applied over each boil. *Rajah Boil.* See *Carbuncle.*

Bones, Scrofulous Affections of. Give Fish Liver Oil (138).

Bowel, Lower, Descent of. The protruded part having been carefully washed, should be replaced by gentle pressure with the hand: should there be any difficulty in doing this, the forefinger well oiled should be pushed up into the anus; and it will, unless the parts be greatly swollen, carry the protruded part in with it. The patient should then remain quiet for some hours in a recumbent posture, and apply cloths saturated with Decoction of Galls (147), or Babúl Bark (9), holding Alum (25*) in solution. Subsequently enemas of the above solutions, or others containing Sulphate of Iron (179), act usefully in constringing the parts and preventing a return of the accident. In weak, debilitated subjects, Confection of Pepper (300) proves very serviceable. The bowels should be kept open by mild aperients, of which Sulphur and Cream of Tartar (344) is by far the best. All straining at stool should be carefully avoided. A person subject to this accident should wear a pad to keep the parts up.

Chronic Descent of the Bowel in Children may be frequently cured by making the child, when at stool, sit on a seat sufficiently high, so that its feet cannot touch the ground, or have other support by any other means. (Dr. Aitchison.)

Bowels, Spasmodic, and other Painful Affections of. Mild cases generally yield to Omum Water (318*), Lemon Grass Oil (216), or the Infusions of Ginger (155), Dill Seeds (134), or Cloves (105), with or without a single dose of Opium (284). Severe cases require the repetition of the Opium (284) in Omum Water, &c., together with either Hot Water Fomentations (393), Mustard Poultices (251), or Turpentine Stupes (362) externally to the abdomen; followed in protracted cases by an enema of Turpentine (364), or Assafœtida (36). In all cases a dose of Castor Oil is advisable when the pain has abated. *In Children*:— See *Colic*. *For Irregularity of the Bowels*, try Bael Sherbet (45); *in that of Children*, Decoction of Kariyát Leaves (193). *Constipation of*. See *Constipation*. *Bleeding from*. See *Hæmorrhage*.

Breast, Abscess of, in Women. See *Milk Abscess*.

Breathing, Difficulty of, occurring without evident cause or in connexion with a cold, sometimes yields to Camphor and Assafœtida Pills (70), and Turpentine Stupes (362), or Mustard Poultices (247) to the chest. Great relief, especially in the case of children, is often derived from external application of Betel leaves (48), or bags of hot salt. See also *Cough*.

Bronchitis, Chronic. Decoction of Sweet Flag (13), Country Ipecacuanha (370), Assafœtida (37), and Fish Liver Oil (140) internally, with Rice Poultices (322), Croton Liniment (122), and Turpentine Stupes (362) externally, may be used with advantage. The inhalation of the vapour of hot Decoction of Abelmoschus (2) is also serviceable. The temperature of the apartment should be kept as uniform as possible. For the relief of a paroxysm of cough, the fumes of burning Nitre Paper (268) are worthy of a trial in all cases. A blister to the chest often affords great relief.

Bronchocele. See *Goitre*.

Bruises. See *Sprains.*

Buboes often subside under a non-stimulant diet, perfect rest in the recumbent posture, and the continued application of Sal Ammoniac Lotion (332), the bowels being at the same time carefully regulated. Should matter form, treat as Abscess (*which see*). Should ulceration result, apply Borax Lotion (59), Resin Ointment (372), &c., as advised for ulcers. 'Buboes especially of the groin, when not in an inflamed condition, are often immensely benefited by having a smooth stone of two pounds weight or thereabout, laid over them ; this rapidly causes absorption.' (Dr. Aitchison.)

Burning of the Feet in Natives. Apply Henna or Mhíndí Poultice (197) locally, and try Bromide of Potassium, 5 to 10 grains dissolved in water, twice or thrice daily.

Burns and Scalds. As soon after the accident as possible, apply freely to the whole of the burnt surface Lime Liniment (229), or in its absence Jinjili Oil (337), or any other bland Oil, dusting thickly over with Rice Flour; or even with simple Rice Flour without any oil as directed in paragraph 322. The object in each case is to prevent, as far as possible, the access of air to the burnt surface. These first dressings should remain undisturbed for at least twenty-four hours, and should then be repeated in the same, or in a modified form. Subsequent ulcerations should be treated with Ceromel (167) or Resin Ointment (372).

Carbolized Oil or Liniment is advocated by Dr. Aitchison.† Should the injured surface be extensive, the constitution should be supported by liberal diet, tonics, and stimulants, as Brandy Mixture (426) at stated intervals. Any great restlessness or excessive pain may require a dose of Opium at bed time (283). N.B. Whenever the burn is in the neighbourhood of a joint, or in the neck, it is important that the parts should be kept in a straight or stretched position, otherwise contraction is apt to result during the healing process.

Cancer. To relieve the pain and restlessness, give Opium (283) or Tincture of Datura (128). *To correct the fœtor of the discharge,* apply relays of Charcoal Poultices (91), cleansing the ulcer each time the poultice is changed with Borax Lotion (59). N.B. On the smallest suspicion of a cancer forming, no time should be lost in placing the case under regular medical care.

Carbuncle, 'Rajah Boil' of the Natives. The treatment of the early stages is similar to that for Abscess

† Dr. A.'s directions are as follows, 'Employ a Liniment of Carbolic Acid, one part Acid to 10 of Oil, carefully mixed; apply this freely over the burnt or scalded surface, cover the whole with a thick piece of cotton wool, and apply a bandage over all. On no account change the cotton dressing unless there is any disagreeable odour. If the dressing is becoming dry and thus causing irritation, take off the bandage and moisten the cotton wadding thoroughly with the same Liniment without moving it. On no account allow water to come in contact with the injured part.'

(*ante*); only if leeches are deemed necessary, they should be placed round the edge and not on the hardened surface. When ulceration sets in, the Toddy Poultice (355) is useful in stimulating to healthy action; and the removal of the slough is greatly accelerated by the daily practice of Irrigation (395). Turpentine Ointment (367) or Petroleum (416) also prove useful in this stage. Should there be much fœtor, apply Charcoal Poultices (91) and the Borax Lotion (59) as advised in *Cancer*. Opium (283) may be necessary to relieve pain and give rest. When the slough has come away, the ointments advised in paragraphs 367 and 372, or Ceromel (167), may be used as dressing. A generous animal diet, with a daily portion of stimulants, should be allowed, and tonics as Chiretta (98, 99), or Country Sarsaparilla (163), administered. Whenever practicable, the case should be placed under proper surgical care, as incisions are often necessary for the removal of the slough.

Cassava Root, Poisoning by. Give Lime Juice (234).

Castor Oil Seeds, Poisoning by. Give Lime Juice (234).

Cataract. Datura (128).

Catarrhs or Colds may often be cut short at the outset by a draught of hot Infusion of Ginger (156) or White Wine Whey (428) at bed-time, and covering the body well, so as to produce copious perspiration. A Vapour Bath (396) will answer the same purpose. To relieve feverishness give Solution of Nitre (364),

Decoction of Abelmoschus (2), and Country Ipecacuanha (370). Inhalation of the fumes of burning Turmeric (359) manifestly relieves troublesome congestion or fulness of the head, nose, &c. See also *Cough*.

Caterpillars' Hairs, to Extract. Some Indian Caterpillars are armed with a thick hairy covering, and if these come in contact with the skin the hairs are apt to pierce the cuticle, and by their presence create great pain, irritation, &c. To extract them the following ingenious plan, devised by Dr. Alexander Grant, late Bengal Medical Service, is said to be very effectual. Take a lock of human hair, tie firmly with thread about one-eighth of an inch from the cut end, so as to form a short, firm, even brush, not however to be used as such, but as forceps. This held between the thumb and forefinger, is allowed to descend perpendicularly and uncompressed among the caterpillar hairs. When the two sets of hairs are commingled, the brush is compressed as forceps are, and drawn straight up, bringing the hairs with it, and so on until all the hairs are pulled out.

Centipedes, Bites of. See *Bites, Venomous.*

Chest, Pains in, during Fevers. See *Fevers.*

Childbirth. See *Labours.*

Children, Debility of. To relieve pallor and wasting, give Country Sarsaparilla (163), and Fish Liver Oil (139), with generous diet, and gentle out-door exercise. A change of air will often do more good than medicine. *Constipation of,* See *Constipation. Convulsion of,* See *Convulsions. Colic of,* See *Colic. Coughs of,* See *Coughs. Diarrhœa of,* See *Diarrhœa. Difficulty of Breathing,* See *Breathing, Difficulty of.*

Cholera. To check the premonitory diarrhœa or purging, give the Alum Powders (26), or Alum with Infusion of Sweet Flag (13), or Omum Water (319); should these not succeed in checking it, try a few of the Compound Pepper Pills (299), but it is unadvisable to continue them long on account of the large proportion of Opium which they contain (285).† Should the disease progress, Dr. Ayre's plan of treatment (285*), if the ingredients are at hand, should be pursued, together with the persevering use of Lemon Grass Oil (216) and Omum Water (318), for the purpose of checking the vomiting, and stimulating the system. For the latter purpose also give an ounce (two table spoonfuls) of the Brandy Mixture (426) every half hour or oftener, unless Champagne or other sparkling wine is available, this being decidedly the best form of stimulant in these cases—only

† One of the most useful forms of Cholera Pills, which should be commenced at the earlier stages when the purging sets in, is composed of 24 grains of Acetate of Lead, and two grains of Opium, made into a mass with a few drops of Honey, and divided into eight pills. Of these one may be given every hour or half hour, according to the urgency of the symptoms, till the whole eight have been taken; but this number should not be exceeded, in consequence of the quantity of Opium they contain. Each pill may be taken in a wine glassful of Omum Water.

it must be given in moderation at stated periods; more harm than good is done by over-stimulation. The patient should be encouraged to drink plentifully of *cold* water, iced if possible; though the first draught or two may be rejected, it will soon be retained if persevered in. Chicken broth, or Lime Water and Milk, may also be given plentifully as a drink. The other accessories to the above are Mustard Poultices (251) or Turpentine Stupes (363) over the heart (left side of the chest), bags of hot sand or salt to the spine, feet, and legs, and diligent friction with the hand or hot towels. At the same time the patient should not be moved about more than can be possibly helped. N.B. During an epidemic of Cholera impress upon everybody the necessity of applying for medicines directly they feel unwell or have the slightest purging; those who come thus early for treatment stand a much better chance of recovery than those who delay even a few hours. Here time is of the most vital importance.

Chorea, St. Vitus's Dance. Fish Liver Oil (141), Infusion of Jatamansi (184), and Sulphate of Iron (177), alone or in combination, according to circumstances, are worthy of a trial. N.B. This, as well as other nervous affections, is often due to intestinal worms: attention should therefore be paid to this point. (See *Convulsions.*)

Cocculus Indicus, Poisoning by. Having emptied the stomach by an emetic of Sulphate of Copper (117) or Mustard (246), give copious draughts of Decoction of Galls (152), followed by a full dose of Castor Oil to carry off any of the poison which may have passed into the intestines. Brandy or other stimulants are required should there be great depression or exhaustion.

Colds. See *Catarrhs.*

Colic in Adults is to be treated in a manner described in Spasmodic Affections of the Bowels. *The Colic of Children,* usually connected with flatulence, generally yields to Omum Water (318*), Infusion of Dill (134), with or without Assafœtida (36), and a Hot Bath (387), followed by a dose of Castor Oil.

Constipation. For the immediate relief of this, aperients are required. Castor Oil (84) and Senna (336, 337) are best adapted for children and delicate females; Aloes (18, 19) for women suffering from irregularity or suspension of the menstrual discharge; Myrobalans (256) and Kaladana (187) for otherwise healthy adults; and Croton Pills (120) or Croton Oil when strong and speedy purgation is indicated. *The Constipation of Hysterical Females* is best treated by Aloes and Assafœtida Pills (19); *Habitual Constipation,* by Aloes, as directed in Paragraph 20, or by Sulphur (344); *that of Children* by Fish Liver Oil (139), together with the use of oatmeal as an article of diet. A remedy for habitual constipation in children, as well as in adults, is to be sought for in tonics rather than in purgatives; the repeated use of the latter lays the foundation of great subsequent mischief. N.B. The practice of native ayahs of inserting a piece of tobacco stem into the anus of young children to relieve constipation, cannot be too strongly reprobated.

Consumption, Pulmonary (Phthisis). The persevering use of Fish Liver Oil (138) is chiefly to be relied upon, with or without Lime Water and Milk (226) as an ordinary drink. *As a preventive* sponge the chest daily with diluted Vinegar (378). Mustard Poultices (247) or Croton Liniment (122) to the chest sometimes gives relief to *the Cough and Difficulty of Breathing,* as does the inhalation of the vapour of Hot Water (390) or Decoction of Abelmoschus (3). *For the Diarrhœa,* try the Alum Powders (26), or Sulphate of Copper (110). *For the excessive Perspirations,* sponge the chest with Vinegar (378). *For the Sore Mouth or Fissures of the Tongue,* apply Borax (55), or Alum (29). *For Bleeding from the Lungs* try some of the means mentioned in *Hæmorrhage, Internal.*

Convulsions in Adults, arising without evident cause, are best treated by cold Affusion (386), Mustard Poultices (248), or Turpentine Stupes (363) to the feet and legs, and a strong purgative, as Croton Pills (120), Croton Oil (121), or Kaladana (187). If the patient be unable to swallow, a Turpentine enema (364) may be used. *When the Convulsions are due to poisons, &c., taken into the stomach,* an emetic of Mustard (246) or Sulphate of Copper (117) should precede all other measures. *In the Convulsions of Labours,* Turpentine Stupes (363) or Mustard Poultices (248) should be applied to the extremities, and Evaporating Lotion

(380) to the head, whilst Camphor and Calomel Pills (73), or Borax and Cinnamon (58), are given internally. A Turpentine enema (364) may also prove useful. *The Convulsions of Children* are best treated with a Hot Bath (387), and a full dose of Castor Oil (84), preceded by one or two grains of Calomel when at hand, or a dose or two of Assafœtida Mixture (36).† When the child is very much exhausted, a few drops of Brandy, three to six, or more, according to age, are often most useful. Convulsions of early childhood are frequently connected with teething, hence lancing the gums is often of essential benefit.

N.B. Convulsions and nervous affections occurring in Natives and Anglo-Indians are very frequently due to the presence of worms in the intestines; their existence may perhaps be unsuspected, or even denied; hence in all cases which resist ordinary treatment, it is advisable to give a trial to one or more of the

† *In the Convulsions of Infancy and Childhood*, especially when the cause is obscure, unconnected with teething, &c., Bromide of Potassium is often more serviceable than any other remedy, in doses of a quarter of a grain for a child under six weeks of age, half a grain under three months, one grain above that age to nine months, and one grain additional for every year up to three or four years of age. And these doses may be safely repeated every two, three, or four hours until the convulsions subside. The smaller doses may be obtained with exactitude by dissolving, say, one grain of the Bromide in four tea spoonfuls of water, and giving one, two, or three spoonfuls, or the whole quantity, as one quarter, one half, one third, or one grain respectively is required. It is worthy of a fair trial in all cases which resist ordinary means, but should not be used to the exclusion of the hot bath and careful regulation of the bowels.

remedies recommended for *Worms*, especially those for the *Lumbricus or Round Worm*, which is so extensively prevalent in India.

Corns are best treated by immersion in hot soap and water, paring off the hardened cuticle and wearing a piece of thick plaster, with or without a hole in the centre, to ward off the pressure and friction. *For Corns between the Toes* nothing is more effectual than a piece of thick blotting-paper worn so as to protect the opposing surfaces: it should be renewed daily. If only ordinary thin blotting-paper be available, two folds are advisable.

Corrosive Sublimate, Poisoning by. See *Mercurial Salts, Poisoning by.*

Coughs. Try Sal Ammoniac (329) and Country Ipecacuanha (370); with Rice Poultices (322) or Mustard Poultices (247), Turpentine Liniment (366), or Camphorated Opium Liniment (291) externally, and the inhalation of the vapour of Hot Water (390) or Decoction of Abelmoschus (2). If severe, a blister (349, 350) to the chest may be necessary. *In Chronic cases, especially when attended with much expectoration and debility,* give Fish Liver Oil (140). *In Spasmodic Coughs,* violent paroxysms may be relieved by inhaling the fumes of Nitre Paper (268), or by smoking Datura (129). *For the Cough of Old Age,* Cubebs (126) is worth a trial. *For the Cough of Childhood,* Syrup of Country Liquorice (6), Assafœtida (37), Honey and Vinegar (166), and Fish Liver Oil, may be resorted to according to circumstances. Camphor Liniment (70), Mustard Poultices (247), or bags filled with hot salt, or better still, Betel Leaves (48), applied externally, tend to *relieve difficulty of breathing in these cases.* Sponging the chest with Vinegar is thought to lessen the liability to attacks (378).

Coup de Soleil. See *Sunstroke.*

Croton Oil Seeds, Poisoning by. See Parag. 234.

Croup. Sulphate of Copper (111) as an emetic, and Hot Water Stupes (390) externally, are valuable accessories in the treatment of this disease.

'The best and readiest emetic,' writes Dr. Aitchison, 'is a pinch of Ipecacuanha powder placed dry at the back of the child's tongue. This usually acts instantaneously, so be prepared for the emergency. Sponges dipped in extremely hot water, then rinsed out, and continuously applied over the throat, will often check a coming attack. Poultices are useful, but are apt to do much harm if allowed to become cold. Mustard poultices should not be applied, as without due care they are apt to make the skin tender, and thus prevent the use of hot fomentations.'

Datura, Poisoning by swallowing the seeds of, &c., is to be treated in the manner directed for Opium poisoning. *Where Insensibility arises from the Inhalation of the Fumes,* Cold Water Affusion (386) in the open air often succeeds in removing it at once. The patient should be aroused by any or all of the means enumerated in poisoning by Opium. The nervous symptoms may continue for two or three days, and yet recovery follow.

Debility, Constitutional, requires the use of the following tonics, either alone or combined: Chiretta (98, 99*), Sweet Flag Root (12), Country Sarsaparilla (163), Kariyát (191), Ním-Bark (260), or Gulancha (352). *When attended with Anœmia or great pallor of the surface, especially of the inner surface of the eyelids and tongue,* Sulphate of Iron (174) is indicated. The efficacy of all these remedies is increased by a liberal animal diet, and gentle exercise in the open air. *Debility after Fevers.* See *Fevers.*

Delhi Sores. The Borax Ointment (59) is strongly recommended. See also *Ulcers.*

Delirium generally is best treated by Evaporating Lotion (380) to the head, the Mustard Foot Bath (248), or Turpentine Stupes (363) to the extremities and a strong purgative; *for that occurring in Fevers,* see *Fevers.*

Delirium Tremens. *To relieve sleeplessness and anxiety,* give Opium and Camphor (283), or better still, Bromide of Potassium, as advised in *Sleeplessness in Head Affections.* See that article. Try also the Mustard Foot Bath (248, 249), or the Wet Sheet (398). *To support the strength,* give Brandy Mixture (427*) and a nourishing diet.

Diabetes. Vapour baths (396) in the early stages, Alum Whey (27) and Lime Water (226) internally, with Opium (288), at bed-time, prove occasionally useful as palliatives. Their operation is assisted by a full animal diet, with a diminished quantity of rice and other farinaceous food, and by warm clothing. Use Lemonade as a drink (232).

Diarrhœa. In the early stages, especially if attended with heat of skin, &c., give Country Ipecacuanha (369) and Ispaghúl seeds (304), with a mild aperient, as Castor Oil, if there is reason to think that the attack arises from crude, undigested food in the intestines. The Acetate of Lead and Opium Pills advised for Cholera are often very successful in these cases. One may be given every two or three hours, or oftener, according to the urgency of the symptoms; they are especially useful in *Epidemic Diarrhœa. In the advanced stages or in Chronic Diarrhœa* try Sulphate of Copper (110), Catechu (88), Alum (26), or one of the following: Decoction of Babúl Bark (9), Infusion of Sweet Flag (13), Bael (44), Butea Gum (62), Galls (146), Decoction of Pomegranate (312), and Omum Water (318), with or without the addition, in each case, of a small portion of Opium (289). Turpentine Stupes (363) to the abdomen are useful if much pain is present. *Where the disease is apparently of malarious origin or connected with periodic Fevers of any kind*, Quinine (three to five grains twice or thrice daily) should be associated with whatever other remedies are being employed. Try also Warm Water Enemas (393). *When connected with Acidity of the Stomach*, give Lime Water (222). *When caused by Over-eating or by Indigestible Food*, follow up an emetic of Mustard

(246) or Country Ipecacuanha (368), to unload the stomach, by Omum Water (318), and subsequently by a dose of Castor Oil. Capsicum (79) is thought to be specially useful *in Diarrhœa arising from the use of putrid food, e.g., fish.* *The Diarrhœa of Children* often yields to a dose of Castor Oil, if given early; if not, one of the following may be tried: Acorus or Sweet Flag (13*), Bael (44), Catechu (88), Sulphate of Copper (110), Sulphate of Iron (181*), Saccharated Solution of Lime (222), or Ispaghúl Seeds (304). Omum Water (318) may be advantageously combined with any of the above. *The Diarrhœa which precedes Cholera.* See *Cholera.* N.B. In all cases of diarrhœa the food should be mild and unirritating, thick Arrowroot (423) being the best suited for the purpose, and in all obstinate or chronic cases, a flannel bandage should always be worn round the abdomen.

Dropsy occurring in the young and vigorous is best treated at the outset by strong purgatives, as Croton Pills (120) or Oil (121), or Kaladana (187), followed by medicines which increase the flow of urine, as Decoction of Asteracantha (39), Infusion of Moringa (237), Mustard Whey (250), or Infusion of Pedalium (297), with which Nitre (269) or Sal Ammoniac (331), may be combined as circumstances require. The Vapour Bath (396), twice a-week, proves useful in recent cases, where the patient is strong enough to bear it. Where the patient is very debilitated and anæmic (174), Sulphate of Iron (178) should be tried.

Drunkenness. After a debauch, a Mustard emetic (246) proves most useful in unloading the stomach of any spirit remaining in it. A few drops, six to twelve, of Liquor Ammoniæ in water subsequently given, are often of signal success. Strong Coffee, 'café noir,' is also most useful. *To allay the subsequent cravings for drink* try Omum Water (320).

Dysentery. In the early stages give Country Ipecacuanha (369) and Ispaghúl Seeds (304), or Sesamum leaves (Foot-note, p. 139), with or without Opium (289*), and apply Hot Fomentations to the abdomen and Leeches to the verge of the anus (211); the latter tend much to relieve the pain and straining, as do also Opiate enemas (289).† *When of malarious*

† The treatment of Acute Dysentery by large doses of Ipecacuanha, re-introduced into practice in 1858 by Dr. Docker, is acknowledged by the most experienced authorities to be far more effectual than any other. It consists, in the main, of administering, as early in the disease as possible, 25 to 30 grains of Ipecacuanha, in as small a quantity of fluid as possible, premising half an hour previously 25 to 30 drops of Laudanum. The patient should keep perfectly still in bed, and abstain from fluids for at least three hours. If thirsty, he may suck a little ice, or may have a tea spoonful of cold water. It is seldom, under this management, that nausea is excessive, and vomiting is rarely troublesome, seldom setting in for two hours after the medicine has been taken. Mustard Poultices (247) or Turpentine Stupes (362) should be applied to the abdomen. In from eight to ten hours, according to the urgency of the symptoms and the effect produced by the first dose, Ipecacuanha in a reduced dose should be repeated, with the same precautions as before. The effects of this treatment are soon manifest and surprising; the griping and straining subside, the motions quickly become feculent, blood and slime

origin or when occurring in the course of periodical Fevers, Quinine (three to five grains twice or thrice daily) should form part of whatever other treatment is being followed. *In the advanced stages, or when it passes into Chronic Dysentery,* apply Turpentine Stupes (362) to the abdomen, and give Sulphate of Copper (110), Bael (44), Infusion of Kariyát (191), Decoction of Pomegranate Rind (312), or Sal Ammoniac (331). When an aperient is required, give Sulphur and Cream

disappear; and often, after profuse action of the skin, the patient falls into a tranquil sleep and awakes refreshed. The treatment may require to be continued for some days, the medicine being given in diminished doses, care being taken to allow a sufficient interval to admit of the patient taking some mild nourishment suited to the stage of the disease. As the disease abates, the dose should be reduced. It is well, however, to administer 10 or 12 grains at bed-time for a night or two, after the stools are, to all appearance, healthy. Fomentations or Turpentine Stupes to the abdomen, lessen griping and diminish suffering. If a little diarrhœa without the dysenteric odour remain, it may be checked with a little astringent mixture, with or without Opium. Astringents in any shape during the acute stage are not only useless, but dangerous.—(Dr. Maclean.) To sum up, it appears—1. That acute dysentery is more successfully and speedily treated by large doses of Ipecacuanha than by other means. 2. That it is more effectual in the acute than in the chronic forms. 3. That large doses, such as are mentioned above, may be given with perfect safety, without fear of ill effects; and 4. That it is less successful with the natives of India than with Europeans. In the acute dysentery of natives, small doses, *e. g.*, from six to eight grains thrice daily, so as to keep up a slight degree of nausea, short of actual vomiting, seem to answer better than the large doses mentioned above. It may be advantageously combined with Opium, from quarter to half grain with each dose.

of Tartar (344) or Castor Oil, with the addition of a small portion of Opium. *For the Dysentery of Natives,* Decoction of Sweet Flag (13), Galls (146), Mudar (243), Opium (289), and Decoction of Pomegranate Rind (312), seem best suited. *For the Chronic Dysentery of Children* the Saccharated Solution of Lime (222), Bael (44), Sulphate of Copper (110), or Sulphate of Iron (181), are indicated. See also *Diarrhœa of Children.* N.B. In all cases of dysentery the food should be mild and unirritating, and a flannel bandage worn round the abdomen. Soups containing mucilage of Abelmoschus (2) prove useful.

Dysmenorrhœa. See *Menstruation, Painful.*

Dyspepsia. See *Indigestion.*

Ear, Discharges from, in Scrofulous Subjects. Syringe the ear daily with Lime Water (225), or tepid water, or milk and water, and give Fish Liver Oil internally (138). *Buzzing or Noises in the Ear* often depend upon an accumulation of wax in the outer passage; to remove this and effect a cure, all that is necessary in many cases is to insert a drop or two of sweet oil for an hour or two, and then to syringe the ear well out with tepid water or soap and water, and repeat the same twice or thrice daily. This also sometimes relieves *Ear-Ache:* if not, use Opium as directed in Para. 292.

Elephantiasis. The paroxysms of fever which accompany this disease are to be treated in the manner directed for Intermittent Fever (*infra*). The only means of arresting the progress of the disease is to remove permanently from a locality in which it is endemic or prevalent, to another situated at least ten miles distant from the sea-coast; the higher and drier the site, the better.

Epilepsy sometimes improves under Fish Liver Oil (241); its use may be combined with Sulphate of Copper, in doses of a quarter of a grain twice or thrice daily. For this purpose, dissolve two grains in one ounce of Omum Water; of this, the dose is a teaspoonful.† See also remarks at the end of *Convulsions* in this Index.

Exhaustion from Hæmorrhage after Fevers or other causes, give Brandy Mixture (426).

Eyes, Affections of. Datura (128). *For 'Country Sore Eye,'* apply Alum, as directed in Paragraph 23, and Decoction of Turmeric (360) to relieve the burning sensation. Try also Solution of Sugar (409). *For other forms of Ophthalmia, attended with copious discharge*, try Sulphate of Copper (113). *To relieve great pain and intolerance of light*, use Opium locally (292). *Blows on the Eye:* Alum Poultice (24), followed by Sal

† Far superior to all other remedies for *Epilepsy* is Bromide of Potassium in doses of 10 to 15 grains, in a wine glassful of water, thrice daily. Should the disease not yield to these doses they may be gradually increased to double or even treble these quantities. The earlier in the disease this remedy is resorted to the greater are its chances of success; and as a general rule it proves more useful when the fits are severe and frequent, and occur mainly in the day-time than in the milder attacks which come only at night. In all cases it is worthy of a fair trial.

Ammoniac Lotion (332), to remove discoloration. *Particles of Lime in the Eye* may be dissolved and removed by dilute Vinegar (382). *Particles of Dirt, &c.*, may often be speedily dislodged and removed by drawing the upper eyelid well over the under one as far as possible, for a few seconds. This simple plan is often successful when others fail. If this fail, try Solution of Sugar (409). Fresh Plantain Leaf (307) forms an excellent shade for the eyes in all affections of those organs.

Face-Ache, Neuralgic or Rheumatic. Sal Ammoniac (326), Sulphate of Iron (177), or Fish Liver Oil (141) internally; and Datura (130), and Mustard (252), or Ginger (157) Poultices locally, are measures which used conjointly often prove successful. *When periodical*, Cinchona Febrifuge (402*).

Fainting generally yields to dashing cold water over the face and neck (386), and applying strong smelling salts to the nostrils; when partially recovered, Omum Water (318) or Assafœtida (35) may be given, or should there be much exhaustion, a dose of Brandy Mixture (426).

Fevers, Ardent or Continued. In most cases it is advisable to commence with a purgative of Kaladana (187), Castor Oil (84), or Myrobalans (256), or if the patient be a strong adult, a Croton Pill (120); after its operation, the Solution of Nitre (264) may be given; and Decoction of Abelmoschus (2), Lemonade (232), or Tamarind Infusion (346), *to allay the thirst and cool the system.* A very useful and refreshing drink in all fevers, especially if there is irritability of the stomach is a mixture of equal parts of Milk and Soda Water; with the addition of a piece of ice if procurable. Sucking small pieces of ice, also, allays thirst and cools the system; for this latter purpose, also, sponging the surface with Water (385) or diluted Vinegar (376) may be employed. The diet should consist chiefly of Rice Conjee (322), and other farinaceous articles, and the apartment should be kept cool and well ventilated. *To relieve Headache or great fulness of the head,* apply constantly Evaporating Lotion (380), or Nitre Lotion (265), or if these fail to afford relief, Hot Water Fomentations (393). Leeches to the temples or nape of the neck (209), and Mustard Poultices to the feet (248), may also be necessary in severe cases. *For any severe or acute pain arising in the chest or abdomen,* Leeches, (209) over the seat of pain should be applied, but if these fail, try a Blister (349). *For Vomiting and Irritability of Stomach,* give Lime Water (223), or else give Hot Water as a drink (385), and apply Mustard Poultices (251)—*For Bilious Diarrhœa accompanying,* use Warm Water Enemas (393). *For Sore Throat or Fissures of the Tongue,* apply Borax (55), or Alum (29); *for Dryness of the Mouth and Fauces,* sucking sliced limes, or, better still, pine apples, generally suffices. *In the advanced stages, when great exhaustion, delirium, &c.,* are present, give Camphor (74) and Brandy Mixture (426) internally, and apply Turpentine Stupes (363) to the extremities; Turpentine Enemas (364) are also valuable in this condition. *For subsequent*

Debility, and during Convalescence, give one of the following tonics: Chiretta (98), Atís (42), Bonduc (52), Kariyát (191), Ním Bark (260), Gulancha (352–3), or Cinchona Febrifuge (402). A combination of Chiretta and Sweet Flag Root (12), or Chiretta Wine (99) is perhaps best suited for this purpose. A liberal animal diet should be allowed. N.B. Throughout the attack it is essential to keep the bowels properly regulated.

Fever, Intermittent or Ague, and Remittent or Jungle Fever. Commence with an aperient, as in Fever (*ante*), and should the stomach be foul, give an emetic of Country Ipecacuanha (368). *In the cold stage*, cover the body well up, give Infusion of Ginger (69), and place bags containing hot sand or hot salt along the spine. *In the hot stage*, give plentifully of Lemonade (232), Solution of Nitre (264), and adopt generally the other measures advised above in Fever. *In the sweating stage*, do nothing but protect the surface from cold draughts of air or cold winds. In the intermission or periods between the paroxysms, give one of the following—Atís (42), Bonduc Nut (52), Chiretta (98), Sulphate of Iron (175), Ním Bark (260), or Gulancha (352). When one fails another may succeed; when each fails given singly, they will sometimes prove effectual given in combination. They are all greatly inferior in efficacy to Quinine † and Cinchona Febrifuge

† In mild, ordinary, uncomplicated cases of *Intermittent Fever*, all that is required, due attention being paid to state of the bowels and secretions, is to administer Quinine in doses of from three to five grains, so that 10 or 12 grains be taken in the intermissions between the paroxysms. It is best given in

(401, 403). *For these Fevers in Natives,* Galls with Chiretta, and Sweet Flag Root (12), have been favourably spoken of. *Swelling of left side after Ague,* See *Spleen, Enlargement of.*

solution, in water or coffee. In the severer forms, or even in ordinary cases, Professor Maclean, of the Netley Hospital, has proposed a treatment which appears very judicious, and which in his hands has for years proved very successful. It consists in administering 30 grains in three equal doses during the period of intermission; the first dose, in solution should be given towards the close of the sweating stage, and the last about as far as can be calculated, an hour before the next anticipated paroxysm. Should there be much irritability of the stomach, it should be given in enema in doses of 15 grains in place of 10 grains. After the paroxysm has by this means been arrested, a moderate degree of cinchonism, *i.e.*, giddiness, buzzing in the ears, flashing before the eyes, &c., should be maintained for some days, by giving three or four grains in solution every four hours. In cases where the fever returns at the first lunar period, as it is apt to do, the patient a day or two previously, should be brought under the influence of Quinine, which should be maintained until the time is past. Should it fail to influence the fever, attention should be directed to the state of the liver and bowels. When from any cause it cannot be given internally, trial may be made with it applied endermically; the experiments of Dr. Guastamacchia and others tending to prove that it becomes absorbed into the system through the skin, and operates as an antiperiodic almost as certainly as when given internally. He dissolved eight grains in half an ounce of spirit, and rubbed first one-half, and after the interval of a quarter of an hour, the second half along the spine. When this was done at the commencement of the cold fit, it very often prevented even a single recurrence. Dr. Daunt also bears testimony to this method in the fevers of South America.

In Remittent and Jungle Fever, Quinine is a remedy of the highest value, but its exhibition requires more caution and discrimination than in simple intermittents. Dr. Maclean's

Fits. See *Convulsions, and Hysterical Affections.*

Flatulence, and Flatulent Colic. Give Omum Water (318*), Lemon Grass Oil (216), Infusion of Ginger (155), or of Jatamansi (184); with Mustard Poultices

treatment appears to be worthy of every attention. After premising, in most cases, a cathartic, immediately on the first signs of remission, he administers a full dose of Quinine, 10 grains, often 15, sometimes 20 grains, never exceeding that dose, and not deterred by the presence of headache or a foul tongue, nor because the remission is slight or imperfectly marked; and this dose he repeats every second hour until 30 or 35 grains have been taken before the hour of the expected exacerbation. Should the stomach be too irritable to bear it, it should be given in enema in large doses (20 grains). As soon as the second remission appears, it must be given as before until full cinchonism or distinct abatement of the disease occurs. During the remission the patient should have mild farinaceous diet, milk, chicken-broth, &c.; as soon as gastric irritability subsides, beef tea should be given, and on the first sign of exhaustion, nourishment and stimulants should be resorted to at short intervals. With regard to the administration of Quinine during exacerbations, Dr. Maclean is of opinion that in the adynamic forms of fever, as met with in some parts of India, and in neglected or mismanaged cases, where depletion has been carried too far, and the fever assumes more of a low, continued type, it may be given at any period irrespective of remission. Here it requires to be conjoined with the assiduous use of support and stimulants at short intervals.

As a preventive of Malarious Fever, the power and value of Quinine have been proved beyond a doubt. Every person engaged in forests, swamps, or low, malarious sites, should be provided with a stock of it, and four grains of it in a cup of hot coffee should be taken the first thing in the morning or in a glassful of wine later in the day. Even if it should fail, which it rarely does, no harm can result from its use, and it is essential that it should be continued for at least fourteen days after quitting a malarious locality.

(251) and Turpentine Stupes (362) externally; in severe cases an enema of Assafœtida (36), will generally afford relief. See also *Bowels, Spasmodic Affections of. Of Children*, See *Colic.*

Gall Stones. To allay the severe pain attendant on passing, give Opium (284) and a Hip Bath (392).

Genital Organs, Great Irritation of. Try Camphor (72) internally,† and use Borax (57) and Lime Water (224) locally. Sitting over the steam of hot water, or a tepid hip-bath, often affords great relief. When the irritation arises, as it often does, from worms in the intestines, give some of the remedies for *Worms.* Crab-lice, which are very difficult to distinguish on a dark skin, are also a frequent cause; if present, use Kerosine Oil, or other remedy named in Art. *Lice.*

Glands, Enlarged. Apply externally, in the early stages, Sal Ammoniac Lotion (332), Betel Leaves (48), Camphor Liniment (68), or Opium Liniment (291). If matter forms, treat as abscess, and give Fish Liver Oil internally.

Gleet may be treated with Cubebs (125), Galls (149), Gurjun Balsam (160), or Sandal Wood Oil internally, and Alum Injections (30); these last named, however, require great caution, and should not generally be used except under medical supervision.

† In these cases Bromide of Potassium, in doses of eight to ten grains dissolved in water, twice or thrice daily, is well worthy of a trial, especially in females.

Goitre. Give Sal Ammoniac (324), in ten-grain doses, thrice daily, persevering in its use for weeks or months if necessary. Dr. Stevens (*London Med. Record,* June 15th, 1880) obtained signal benefits from it in six cases. Biniodide of Mercury, in the form of Ointment (16 grains of the Biniodide to one ounce of Simple Ointment), is the best local application we possess. Its effects are best produced by exposing the surface on which it has been rubbed to the direct rays of the sun. If this cannot be done, then to the heat of a fire: this, however, is not nearly so efficacious as the solar heat. (Dr. Aitchison.)

Gonorrhœa. After a purgative of Kaladana (187), Myrobalans (256), or Castor Oil, give Nitre (269) with Decoction of Abelmoschus (2), Ispaghúl (305), or Rice Conjee (322), for the purpose of allaying the pain and heat in passing urine. Pedalium (297) is said to be very effectual for this purpose, and should be tried if procurable. Injections of a solution of Sugar (410) are recommended by Dr. Aitchison. When the inflammatory symptoms begin to abate, one of the following should be given:—Cubebs (125*), Gurjun Balsam (160), Sandal Wood Oil (334), or Galls (149). Alum (30*), locally, is of great use in certain cases. *To relieve Chordee* (painful erection at night), Camphor (72) is one of our best remedies.†

† Bromide of Potassium, in doses of 20 to 30 grains, in a wine glassful of water at bedtime, is highly spoken of, as preventing the occurrence of this symptom.

Guinea Worm. On the head of the worm appearing, it should be gently drawn down so as to secure it by rolling it round a small piece of twisted rag, or a thin piece of quill; and Water Dressing (394) applied, or should there be much pain, a Datura Poultice (132). Every day gentle traction should be made, and if this can be done whilst the limb or part is immersed in a running stream or in a chattie of cold water, the extraction is rendered additionally easy. Great gentleness is requisite to prevent the worm breaking, as this accident is followed by inflammation, and the formation of abscesses, which are difficult of healing. See *Abscess.*

Gums, Ulceration and Sponginess of, may be treated with one of the following:—Decoction of Babúl Bark (9), Alum (29*), Catechu (89*), or Lime Juice (231).

Hæmorrhage from Cuts, Wounds, &c. When the blood is of a bright red colour, and comes out in jets, indicating that an artery is wounded, apply first a stream of *cold* water, iced if possible, from a large sponge, which will not only wash away all clots, dirt, &c., but promote contraction of the vessel, and perhaps arrest the bleeding at once. If not, try the fresh juice of the Physic Nut Plant (302*), or Alum (25). If these fail, or are not at hand, at once apply pressure with the finger or fingers upon the exact point from which the blood is found to issue, and there retain for some time, pressing against the bone or hard substance. If the mouth of the bleeding vessel be clearly visible, and the hæmorrhage still continues, it may be pinched up firmly between the finger and thumb, or it may be seized with a pair of pincers or forceps, drawn forward, and a ligature, silk if procurable, passed round it and firmly tied. Not more of the surrounding flesh should be included in the ligature than can be possibly avoided. If none of these plans succeed or are applicable, or if the wound be large and bleeds much, apply pressure to the limb by means of the STICK TOURNIQUET figured below.†

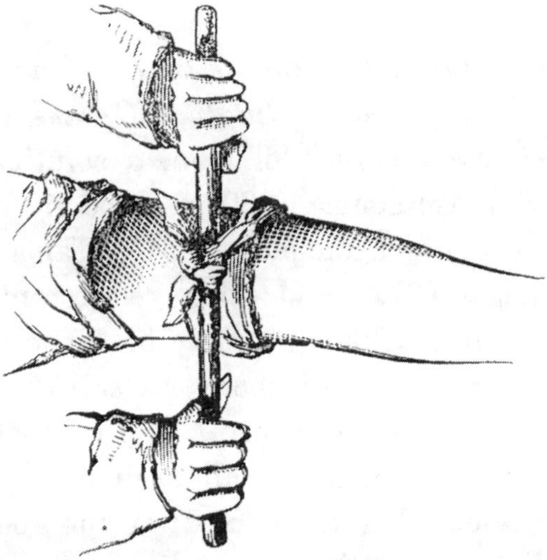

In order to apply this properly, 'tie tightly, at some little distance above the wound, a pocket-handkerchief or cravat once or twice passed round the limb; then, obtaining a piece of tough stick, push it under the handkerchief, and, by turning the stick,

† The above woodcut, and the mode of applying it, is reprinted by permission from *First Help in Accidents*, by Dr. C. H. Schaibe, published by R. Hardwicke, 192 Piccadilly, London. A very useful little book.

twist the handkerchief more and more tightly until the bleeding ceases. As soon as this result has been attained, fasten the stick by another handkerchief round the stick and limb together. This rude tourniquet may save life not unfrequently, by enabling the injured person to be transported even for some distance without fear of further bleeding.' Position is a very important consideration in wounds, the bleeding sometimes being at once arrested by raising the injured limb above the level of the body.

Hæmorrhage from the Lungs, Stomach, Bowels, Kidneys, Uterus, or other Internal Organs, if attended by feverishness and heat of skin, a solution of Nitre (267) or Sal Ammoniac (330) may be given, with the plentiful use of Lemonade (234), Tamarind drink (346), Vinegar (379), and other refrigerants. In the absence of fever, Alum (25) may be given with safety and advantage.† In all these cases perfect rest in a recumbent posture, in a cool, well-ventilated apartment, and the avoidance of all excitement and stimulants, are essential to the success of the above, or any other remedies. In these cases Ice externally applied in bags exercises a marked influence in checking internal hæmorrhage, especially from the lungs. It

† A far more effectual remedy in these cases is the Acetate of Lead in doses of three or four grains, made into a pill with half a grain of Opium, and followed immediately by a draught containing a little vinegar. These pills and draughts may be repeated every three or four hours till the bleeding begins to abate, when the interval between the doses may be lengthened, and the quantities decreased.

should not be kept on sufficiently long to produce a chill. Sucking small pieces of ice is also a useful practice. *Exhaustion from excessive Hæmorrhage* requires Brandy Mixture (426) and other stimulants. *Hæmorrhage after Labours*, See *Labours*. *From Piles*, See *Piles*.

Hæmorrhage from the Nose may generally be checked by one of the following simple means: 1, the application of a cold body, as a key or a piece of ice, to the nape of the neck. 2. By compressing the *opposite* nostril. 3. By standing in the upright position and holding both arms in the air for a few minutes. If these measures fail, recourse may be had to Alum (25*), Sulphate of Copper (116), or Vinegar (379). Should feverishness be present, treat as directed in preceding article.

Hæmorrhage from Leech Bites. See Paragraph 205.

Head, Affections of, where there is determination of blood to the head, with sleeplessness, restlessness, and anxiety. Mustard Bath (249*).

Headaches generally must be treated with reference to their cause. *If from Constipation*, Castor Oil (84), Kaladana (187), Myrobalans (256), or other purgatives. *Of Fever*, hot-water stupes to the nape of the neck (393). *From Bilious derangement*, the same purgatives preceded by a dose of Calomel (three grains) if at hand, and followed by Sal Ammoniac (328*). *Nervous, Hysterical, and Rheumatic Headaches* often yield to Sal Ammoniac (328), persevered in for a few days, and the local use of Camphor Lotion (71*). *From suppression of the Menstrual Discharge,* Leeches to the inner surface of the thighs (210). *From stoppage of bleeding from Piles,* Leeches to the verge of the anus (210); in both these last cases Aloes (19) should be given internally. The other measures occasionally useful are Ginger Poultices (157), Hot Water Fomentations (393), and Mustard Poultices or Mustard Foot-baths (248) to the extremities.

Heart, Palpitations of. See *Palpitations.*

Heartburn often yields to Lime Water (221) given with milk or with Omum Water (317); or with Chiretta (98), if associated with indigestion.

Hepatitis. See *Liver, Inflammation of.*

Hoarseness may be treated by inhalations of the vapour of Hot Vinegar (378*), or Decoction of Abelmoschus (3), by gargles containing Capsicum (78*), Black Pepper (300), or Moringa root (238); by chewing Ginger (158), or allowing a piece of Catechu (89) to dissolve in the mouth.

Hooping Cough. In the early stages regulate the bowels with Castor Oil (84), and give Country Ipecacuanha (370) and Sal Ammoniac (329). As soon as the feverish symptoms have subsided give Alum (28*); should this fail, try Sulphate of Iron (180), with or without Assafœtida (37). If weakness and emaciation exist, or in very obstinate cases, give Fish Liver Oil (140); Mustard Poultices (252) and friction with

Opium Liniment (291) to the spine seem useful in the chronic stage.

Hydrocephalus (*Water on the Brain*) occurring in weak, emaciated children of a scrofulous habit occasionally improves under Fish Liver Oil (139).

Hysterical Affections. Amongst the means useful in controlling these are Assafœtida (35*), Aloes and Assafœtida Pills (19), Jatamansi (184), Omum Water (318), Turpentine enemas (364), and Cold Water Affusion (386).

Indigestion, or Dyspepsia. Tonics, as Chiretta (98, 99*), Sweet Flag Root (12), Country Sarsaparilla (163), and Gulancha (352), combined with stomachics, as Cloves (105), or Cinnamon (102), Capsicum (79), and Omum Water (318*), offer the best prospect of success. *With great increased Secretion,* Butea Gum (62). *With acidity of the Stomach,* Lime Water (221). *With torpidity of the Bowels,* Tincture of Kariyát (192). Without strict attention to diet, and careful regulation of the bowels and other secretions, medicines will have comparatively little effect.

Inflammations, Local or External, require, according to circumstances—Leeches (212), Hot Water Fomentations (393), Water Dressings (394), Evaporating Lotion (380), Sal Ammoniac Lotion (332), and Rice-Flour or Rice Poultices (322) as external applications. A solution of Acetate of Lead (30 grains in a pint of water) forms an excellent soothing lotion, and one which may always be resorted to with safety. The inflamed parts should be kept constantly wet with it by means of moistened cloths.

Influenza. Give plentifully of Solution of Nitre (264), and treat otherwise as described in *Catarrh.*

Insanity. A free action on the bowels by Croton Pill or Croton Oil (120, 121), and the employment of a Mustard Bath (249), are of service in the early stages. No time should be lost in placing the patient under proper medical care.

Insensibility, from whatever cause arising, may be treated in the first instance by the cautious use of Cold Water Affusion (386). A Turpentine enema (364) may also be of service.

Irritation of the Genital Organs. See *Genital Organs.*

Itch. Use Sulphur Ointment (341), or Kerosine Oil (406).

Jaundice. Mild cases often yield to Sal Ammoniac (331), and the free use of purgatives, as Kaladana (187), or Myrobalans (256).

Joints, Injuries or Enlargement of. In the early stages apply lotions of Alum (32), and Sal Ammoniac (332), and subsequently liniments of Camphor (68), and Turpentine (366). *In Chronic Enlargements,* Croton Liniment (122). *Scrofulous affections of the Joints* improve under the use of Fish Liver Oil (138).

Kidneys, Irritable state, and painful affections of. Give plentifully of diluents, as Decoction of Abelmoschus (2), Ispaghúl Seeds (305), or Rice Conjee (322). These with Opium (286), and the use of the Hip Bath (392), are calculated to afford great relief.

Bleeding from, See *Hæmorrhage.*

Labours. Don't interfere unnecessarily; Nature, if left to her own unaided efforts, will accomplish her work in natural uncomplicated labours. Many a woman has lost her life through meddlesome interference on the part of ignorant midwives. *Should the labour be very prolonged, apparently for want of action or power in the womb,* a few doses of Borax and Cinnamon (58) may be given. *For Flooding,* lose no time in resorting to Cold Water Affusion (388), and subsequently use Vinegar locally (379). *To promote the Lochial Discharge, if scanty or arrested,* use Hot Water Fomentations (393). *For After-pains* give a dose of Opium (289). *Convulsions attendant on,* see *Convulsions.*

Leech Bites, to arrest bleeding from, see Paragraph 205.

Leeches, to dislodge from nose and other passages, see Paragraph 206.

Leprosy. Chaulmúgra (94), Gurgun Balsam (161*), Hydrocotyle (169*), or Mudar (242); with these may be advantageously conjoined a prolonged course of Fish Liver Oil (142), or the latter may be tried alone. *For the ulcerations,* poultices of Hydrocotyle (169), or Ním Leaves (261), may be applied with advantage. Opium (283) is often necessary *to relieve pain and* *procure sleep. Whatever other treatment may be adopted, diligent oily frictions over the whole body should form an essential part of it* (161–338). Carbolic Acid promises to prove a most valuable agent in this disease.†

† The treatment of Leprosy by Carbolic Acid Vapour Baths, introduced by Surgeon-General W. Johnston, M.D. (*Times*, June 3rd, 1882), promises good results, and seems well worthy of further trials. All that is required is an ordinary Vapour Bath Apparatus (387), in which the patient sits, and *outside* a chattie or vessel of sufficient size to contain about a quart of liquid, and made with a lengthened curved spout, to fit accurately on an elastic tube of sufficient length as to pass within the vapour-proof envelope. The calibre of this elastic tube should be such as would admit of a continuous and abundant supply of the vapour as it comes from the vessel, resting on a spirit-lamp having a flame sufficient to keep the fluid in the vessel boiling briskly. Prior to the use of this bath, sponging the body with tepid water, holding a piece of washing soda in solution, seems to aid the absorption of the vapour. The Carbolic Acid should be Calvert's Disinfecting fluid, of which a mixture of three or four parts to six or seven of water may be employed. In this Vapour Bath the patient should remain from 30 to 60 minutes (care being taken that a continuous supply of vapour is kept up from outside), and it may be repeated every second or third day according to circumstances. Dr. Johnston informs me that he has never seen any ill effects result from the use of this carbolized aqueous Vapour, even in cases presenting extensive ulcerated surfaces. Some care is requisite in arranging the fold or frill round the aperture through which the head protrudes. 'Were the patient to breathe a little of it,' Dr. J. remarks, 'little injury would result, possibly good, but still, for obvious reasons, he should not be allowed to breathe too much.' Dr. Aitchison directs leprous ulcerations to be treated with a solution of Carbolic Acid (one to seven or ten of Sweet Oil, according to circumstances, and that at the same time the whole body should be rubbed with a weaker solution (1 to 20). This treatment, he remarks, at

Leucorrhœa ('Whites'). Cubebs (125), Nitre (269), Gurjun Balsam (160), or Sulphate of Iron (174*), internally; with vaginal injections containing Babúl Bark (9), Alum (30*), Galls (149) or Lime Water (224), are indicated.

Lice infesting the hair on various parts of the body, especially the pubes, may be destroyed by Cocculus Indicus Ointment (107), Vernonia Seeds (373*b*), or Kerosine Oil (406). Carbolic Acid Wash (1 Acid to 20 Water), applied night and morning, is said to be an effectual remedy.

Lime, Particles of, in the Eye, may be dissolved and removed by dilute Vinegar (382).

Liver, various Affections of, are often greatly benefited by Sal Ammoniac (331). *Enlargement of,* Sal Ammoniac (331*), Pawpaw Juice (296). *Congestion of this organ, especially if arising from over-feeding,* often subsides under a dose of Calomel (three or four grains) at night, followed, in the morning, by an active aperient of Kaladana (187), or Castor Oil (84). Further relief may be obtained by Hot Water Fomentations (393), Turpentine Stupes (362), or Betel Leaves (48), over the region of the liver; if these fail, Leeches to the same site, or to the verge of the anus (211), may afford manifest relief. All, however, will be useless

once removes the horrid odour usually attendant upon these cases, and the patients will readily adopt it, when they distinctly refuse to wash or clean thenselves. With a change in diet, under this treatment these cases, he adds, improve remarkably.

without strict attention to diet, and careful avoidance of all stimulating articles of food and drink.

Lock-jaw, See *Tetanus.*

Loins, pain in the, See *Lumbago.*

Lumbago. Sal Ammoniac (326) internally, with Liniments of Camphor (68), Lemon Grass Oil (217), Opium (291*), Datura Liniment or Poultices (130), or Turpentine (366) externally, often succeed in affording relief. Turpentine Stupes (362) may be tried in severe or obstinate cases.

Lungs, Affections of, See *Coughs, Consumption, and Bronchitis. Bleeding from*, See *Hæmorrhage.*

Maggots on surface of Ulcers, to destroy. Butea Seeds (65).

Maggots in the Nose (*Peenash*), Injections of Oil of Turpentine (363*b*).

Measles. An occasional mild aperient, just sufficient to keep the bowels gently open, the plentiful use of Lemonade (232), or Rice Conjee (322), with or without Nitre (264), together with confinement to bed in a cool well aired apartment, and farinaceous diet for a few days, will generally suffice for recovery in mild, uncomplicated cases. *To allay irritation of the surface*, sponge with diluted Vinegar (376) or Water (385), and dust the surface well over with Rice Flour (322). *Should cough occur*, use some of those means enumerated in Coughs. *The advanced stages, in bad cases, characterized by great exhaustion*, call for the use of Camphor (74), Brandy Mixture (426), and plentiful nourishment.

Menstrual Discharge, Suspension, or Irregularity of (*Amenorrhœa*). Aloes (18), Borax (58), and Sulphate of Iron (174*), alone or combined, may prove serviceable. Try also hip bath with Sesamum Seeds (Footnote, p. 139). *Excessive or long-continued Menstruation*, Alum (25), and Vinegar (379). *When attended with much pain and distress* (*Dysmenorrhœa*), Opium Liniment (291), or Datura Poultice or Liniment (130) to the loins; also hip bath containing Sesamum Seeds, which also may be tried internally (p. 139).

Mercury, Salts of, as Corrosive Sublimate, Poisoning by. If vomiting is not already present it must be excited by a Mustard (246) or other emetic, and the stomach having thus been emptied of any of the poison it may contain, prompt recourse should be had to the white and yolk of raw eggs, which may be given alone or beaten up with rice flour into a paste with milk or water. The after treatment consists in the free use of Rice Conjee and other demulcent drinks, gargles of Alum (29) or Borax (55), to control the salivation; small doses of Opium, should there be much pain, and a milk or farinaceous diet.

Mesenteric Affections of Children are best treated with Fish Liver Oil (139).

Milk, For Increasing the secretion of, Leaves of Castor Oil Plant (85), or of Physic Nut Plant (302);

for Diminishing or Arresting the secretion of, Betel Leaves (49), or flowers of Jasminum Sambac.†

Milk Abscess. In the early stages apply either Sal] Ammoniac Lotion (325), or hot Vinegar stupes (381). Should matter form, treat as *Abscess.*

Mouth, Ulceration of. Try first Sulphate of Copper (112) or Lime Juice (231); if these fail use some of the other remedies mentioned in Art. *Gums, Ulceration and Sponginess of. For Aphthous Ulcerations, i.e. small white specks or ulcers in the mouths of infants and young children,* apply Borax (55*), or Alum (29), or Sulphate of Copper (112); Country Sarsaparilla (163) may at the same time be advantageously given

† This twining plant (Jasminum Sambac, *Aiton*) is cultivated throughout India for the sake of its white fragrant flowers, which are used as votive offerings. The lactifuge property of these flowers was first brought to notice by Mr. J. Wood (*Ph. of India*, p. 136), who speaks of the fact being well known in Madras. Two cases illustrative of their efficacy occurring in the practice of Dr. Mackenzie, C.B., are recorded by Dr. Bidie (*Madras Jour. Med. Sci.*, Aug., 1870). In one case especially, an English lady, all ordinary means had failed to arrest the flow of milk before the flowers were applied; within a few hours they afforded complete relief, and the secretion of milk, which had been unusually copious, was from that time entirely arrested. The results of the other trial were equally satisfactory. For this purpose two, or three handfuls of the fresh flowers bruised are to be applied unmoistened to each breast and renewed once or twice a day. The secretion is sometimes arrested in twenty-four hours, though this generally requires two or even three days (*Wood*). The native names of these flowers are Mogra ka phúl (*Hind., Duk.*), Mogra phúl (*Beng., Guz.*), Malligraip-pú, Mallip-pú (*Tam.*), Mallelú (*Tel.*), Mullup-pú (*Mal.*), Pich-chi-mal (*Cing.*).

internally. *In severer forms* (*Ulcerative Stomatitis*), try Alum (29).

Mumps. Beyond a dose of Castor Oil (84) or Infusion of Senna (336), so as to keep the bowels gently open, little is required beyond keeping the swollen parts covered with a piece of flannel, to protect them from cold draughts of air, and the use of a farinaceous diet for a few days. Should there be much pain, Opium Liniment (291) may be smeared over the surface of the swollen gland at bed-time. Should there be much fever, heat of skin, &c., a few doses of solution of Nitre (264) may be given.

Muscles, Pains in. Give Sal Ammoniac (327) internally, and use Liniments containing Camphor (68), Lemon Grass Oil (217), Opium (291), or Turpentine (366) externally.

Mosquito Bites, to relieve the irritation, try Lime Juice (235), or Vinegar (380).

Nettle Rash, to allay irritation, apply Borax Lotion (57).

Neuralgia. Try Sal Ammoniac (326), or when the pain returns periodically,† Sulphate of Iron (177), or better still Cinchona Febrifuge (402*). Some obstinate

† When Neuralgia of the Head or Face (Tic Douloureux) recurs at stated periods, and is apparently of malarious origin, no remedy is equal to Quinine, which may be given in one large dose (ten grains) shortly before the time when the pain is expected to return. Should it not yield after three or four doses, no advantage will be gained by continuing it. Another plan is to give it in three grain doses in a glass of wine thrice daily between the paroxysms of pain.

cases which resist these and other remedies yield to a course of Fish Liver Oil (141). Among external applications are Datura Liniment or Poultices (130), Lemon Grass Oil (217), Mustard Poultices (253), and the Camphorated Opium (291), or Turpentine Liniment (366).

Nipples, sore or cracked, are benefited by Borax Lotion (56), or Castor Oil (84), or Lime Water (235), locally applied. As a preventive use Infusion of Catechu (90).—[To ensure prevention, the nipple should be carefully washed and dried immediately the child is removed from the breast, and the tissues may be hardened by washing them for a short time before delivery, and after each application to the breast, with a little brandy and water. It is also a useful practice to wear over the nipple a metallic shield, which should be constantly applied when the child is not at the breast.—*Prof. Ringer.*]

Nodes, or Painful Swellings on the Shin-bone. Apply Datura Poultice (130), or other means mentioned in *Tumours, painful.*

Nose, discharge of Matter from. Use injections of Lime Water (225), or tepid Milk and Water, and give Fish Liver Oil (138) internally. *Maggots in,* See *Peenash.*

Nux Vomica, Poisoning by. Follow the treatment advised for poisoning by Cocculus Indicus. Bland Oils, *e.g.*, Til, Cocoa-nut, or Ground-nut Oil, seem to retard its action, hence may be given largely.

Ophthalmia. See *Eyes, Diseases of.*

Opium, Poisoning by. The stomach having been emptied as speedily as possible by an emetic of Sulphate of Copper (117) or Mustard (246), every means should be adopted for rousing the patient; this is to be effected by dashing cold water over the head and chest, walking him quickly about, supported by two attendants in the open air, applying strong salts, &c., to the nostrils, irritating the leg by flagellation with a wet towel, and administering strong coffee, 'café noir,' or if there should be great depression, a little brandy or other stimulant. When the patient can swallow, Decoction of Galls should be given as directed in Paragraph 152. In extreme cases artificial respiration (subsequently described in Appendix, in Art. *Drowning, Recovering from*) must be tried. These measures should be long persevered in; as long as life lasts, hope of recovery is not to be banished.

Pains, Muscular, See *Muscles, Pains in.*

Palpitations of the Heart, Nervous. These may in a great measure be controlled by Assafœtida (35), Camphor (70), or Infusion of Jatamansi (184), either alone or used conjointly. *Palpitations or flutterings in the region of the Heart* which occur in weak, nervous, hysterical subjects, often yield to Bromide of Potassium, in doses of five to ten grains dissolved in water, twice or thrice daily.

Paralysis. Little can be done by non-professionals beyond giving internally Fish Liver Oil (142), alone or with Sulphate of Iron (177) in anæmic or debilitated subjects, and applying irritants, as Croton Liniment (122), Petroleum (414), externally.

Peenash (*Maggots in the Nose*). Oil of Turpentine (363*b*).

Phthisis, See *Consumption, Pulmonary.*

Physic Nut, Poisoning by, See *Croton Seeds.*

Piles. Sulphur (344) internally, and Gall Ointment (148), or astringent enemas, as Decoction of Babúl Bark (9), or Galls (148), suffice in ordinary cases. In old debilitated subjects Confection of Pepper (300) proves very useful. *When inflamed and painful*, the Hip Bath, or sitting over the steam of hot water (391), and the application of a solution of Borax (56) and soft Rice Poultices (322), with or without the addition of Opium (293), give great relief. The Acetate of Lead Solution advised for *Local Inflammations* (p. 219) is peculiarly serviceable in these cases. It may be used cold or warm, as is most agreeable to the patient's feelings. *To control bleeding from*, use Alum (25), or enemas of Sulphate of Iron (179).† Persons subject to Piles will do well

† When bleeding from piles in residents in hot climates has been long continued, it is unadvisable, so long as it remains within moderate bounds, to take any means of arresting it suddenly; the suppression of the discharge having in some instances been known to be followed by congestion and even abscess in the liver, and in others by congestive headaches and determination of blood to the head. It seems to be an effort of nature to relieve the abdominal circulation, which it is unwise to interfere with, unless the discharge be so profuse as to debilitate the patient, and then the object should be rather to moderate, than to arrest it altogether.

to avoid the use of coffee, as this often appears to aggravate the severity of the symptoms. Cleanliness in these cases is of the greatest importance : the parts should be well washed with soap and water after each motion, and if the piles are internal and protrude during evacuations, they should be washed before they are returned.

Pregnancy. For Pains in the Loins use Camphor (68), or Camphorated Opium Liniment (291). *To allay the Vomiting* try Infusion of Cloves (105). A cup of hot coffee and a piece of dried toast should be taken in bed very early in the morning, after which the woman should remain quiet until the usual hour for rising ; by this means the vomiting may often be prevented. When procurable, a glass or two of Sparkling Moselle is often productive of the best effects, allaying the vomiting, and enabling the patient to retain and digest food.

Prickly Heat may in a great measure be relieved by Solution of Borax (57), or Sulphate of Copper (115), and subsequently dusting the surface with Rice Flour (322) or finely-powdered Sandal Wood.

Pyrosis, See *Water Brash.*

Rectum, Stricture and Painful Affections of. Castor Oil (83), Fish Liver Oil (139).

Rheumatism, Acute. Rheumatic Fever may be treated much in the same way as *Ardent or Continued Fever* (*ante*); by confinement to bed in a cool, well-ventilated apartment, farinaceous diet, and abstinence from alcoholic and other stimulants. Nitre (270) should be given freely, with Lemonade (232) as an ordinary drink. The bowels should be carefully regulated, one or two motions procured daily by a dose of Calomel (three or four grains) and Opium (one grain, or even two grains if there should be great pain or restlessness) at bed-time, followed by Infusion of Senna (336), or Castor Oil (84), in the morning. To the swollen and painful joints a strong solution of Nitre (270) should be kept constantly applied; it generally affords great relief; if not, a Datura Poultice or moistened Datura leaf (or Tobacco leaf), applied as directed in Paragraph 130, may be tried.

Rheumatism, Chronic. Here Sal Ammoniac (327) and Country Sarsaparilla (163) promise to be of much use. Chaulmúgra (94), Mudar (242), and Gulancha (352), have been advised, but in long-standing cases more benefit may be expected from Fish Liver Oil (142). The action of the skin may be kept up by Camphor, both internally and in the form of Vapour Bath (69), and by hot Infusion of Ginger (156) at bed-time, and by constantly wearing flannel next to the skin. *Amongst external applications,* Camphorated Opium Liniment (291) and Lemon Grass Oil (217) are the best; the others comprise liniments containing Camphor (68), Croton Oil (122), Oil of Country Nutmeg (274), Petroleum (414), Physic Nut Oil (302), Sulphur (343), and Turpentine (366); Piney Tallow

(373) has been well spoken of. Should one or more joints be specially attacked, make trial of the applications advised in Acute Rheumatism, or of Flour of Sulphur, as directed in Paragraph 343.

Rickets. Fish Liver Oil (138) may be used with great advantage; it may be combined with Sulphate of Iron (177) if the child is weak and anæmic. Lime Water and Milk (222) forms an eligible ordinary drink.

Ringworm. Apply Borax and Vinegar (60), Cassia alata Ointment (81), Unripe Papaw fruit (295), Sulphate of Copper (115), Oil of Turpentine (367), or Kerosine Oil (406).

Saint Vitus's Dance, See *Chorea.*

Salivation. Use gargles of Alum (29), or Borax (55), or try Catechu in substance (89).

Scald Head, See *Ringworm.*

Scarlatina or Scarlet Fever. Commence with an emetic of Country Ipecacuanha (368) or Mudar (241); place the patient in a cool, well-ventilated apartment; give plentifully of Lemonade (232) or Rice Conjee (322) to allay thirst and feverishness, and give Capsicum Mixture (78) internally. *For the sore throat,* inhale the fumes of hot Vinegar (377), and use Capsicum gargle (78). Sponging the surface with diluted Vinegar (376) or Water (385) is attended with great comfort to the patient, and is otherwise beneficial. The advanced stages, complications, and subsequent debility, are treated in the same manner as in Fevers (*ante*).

Sciatica, See *Neuralgia*. Enveloping the whole of the painful limb in the 'Wet sheet' (398) próves sometimes successful when other remedies fail. Quinine in full doses, five to eight grains thrice daily, may be given at the same time.

Scorpions, Stings of. Alum (32), See also *Bites, Venomous.*

Scrofula. Fish Liver Oil (138) proves most useful in cases in which *Abscesses, Ulcers, or Skin Diseases* are present. *Scrofulous Ophthalmia* is also greatly benefited by it. When the patient is debilitated and anæmic, the Oil may advantageously be combined with Sulphate of Iron. Chaumúlgra (94), Hydrocotyle (169), and Lime Water (225), are amongst the remedies occasionally useful. A dose of Opium (283) or Tincture of Datura (128) may be given at night, if the pain or irritation from ulcers or skin disease occasion sleeplessness. A liberal animal diet, gentle out-door exercise, and sea-bathing are valuable adjuncts to the above remedies.

Scurvy. Lime-juice (231) holds the highest rank both as a curative and preventive agent. All acidulous fruits, Lemons, Oranges, Tamarinds (346), &c., may be used with the greatest advantage. As a preventive of Scurvy in jails, &c., Lime Juice and other analogous agents will prove of comparatively little use unless attention is paid to hygienic measures, *e.g.*, the cleanliness, ventilation, dryness of the building, reduction of numbers in cases of overcrowding, and the use of a liberal and wholesome diet, containing a large proportion of fresh vegetables.† *Diarrhœa of*, give Bael (44).

Seminal Discharges, Involuntary. Give Camphor (72) at bed-time. When attended with much sexual excitement, a full dose of Bromide of Potassium, 20 to 30 grains in a wine glassful of water at bed-time, is often most serviceable. These discharges being sometimes due to irritation caused by Thread Worm in the lower bowel, attention should be directed to this point. See *Worms*.

Skin Diseases. Country Sarsaparilla (163*), Chaulmúgra (94), or Mudar (242); or where the affection

† A new antiscorbutic called Ám-chur has lately been brought into use amongst our native troops in India, and promises to be a powerful rival to Lime Juice. It consists of green Mangoes, skinned, stoned, cut into pieces, and dried in the sun. According to Dr. Clarke, Deputy Surgeon-General Eastern Frontier District, Ám-chur not only maintains the digestive energy of the men, but its use amongst troops, where neither a variety of food nor vegetables is obtainable, commends itself strongly as a result of practical experiment to the military authorities. One ration should be half an ounce, which would be equivalent for an ounce of good Lime Juice. (*British Med. Jour.*, Sept. 30, 1882.) Another antiscorbutic well worthy of attention, especially as an article of diet on long voyages, consists of Dried or Preserved Bananas. When carefully prepared, they are agreeable to the taste, much resembling dried figs, of small cost, and will keep good for a lengthened period.

occurs in debilitated, scrofulous, or leprous individuals, Fish Liver Oil (138) may be given internally. One of the following may at the same time be applied externally: Cassia alata (81), Chaulmúgra (94), Lime Liniment (225), Myrobalan Ointment (257), Sulphur (342), Turpentine (367), Kerosine Oil (405*), or Petroleum (415). The Vapour Bath (396) is often very useful where the skin is hard, dry, and rough. Borax lotion (57) in many instances will allay the irritation.

Sleeplessness in Head Affections. Mustard Bath (249). A full dose of the Bromide of Potassium, 20 to 30 grains in a wine glassful of water, taken at bed time and persevered in for days and weeks, will often be found more effectual and less hurtful than the most powerful narcotics. *From pain attendant on Ulcers, Rheumatism,* &c., Opium (283) or Tincture of Datura (128) at bed time. [N.B.—*Sleeplessness, arising from no evident cause, as bodily pain, mental anxiety, &c., is often dependent on an empty state of the stomach,* and many a sleepless night may be prevented, and many a wakeful hour obviated, by the simple process of eating a few biscuits or a crust of bread before going to bed, or during the night as occasion may require.]

Small Pox. Commence with a mild aperient of Castor Oil (84) or Senna (336), place the patient in a cool, well-ventilated room, and give freely Lemonade (232), Rice Conjee (322), &c., with solution of Nitre

(264); sponge the surface daily with diluted Vinegar (376) or Water (385); and, still further, to *allay irritation*, dust the eruption freely with Rice Flour (322). The Carbolic Acid† treatment promises the best results. With the view of *preventing pitting*, apply Lime Liniment (229). *In the advanced stages, attended with great exhaustion, delirium, &c.*, give Camphor (74), Brandy Mixture (426), and other stimulants, with nutriment. *Subsequent debility and convalescence*, treat as in Fever, *q.v.*

Snake Bites. See Appendix B.

Sneezing, when violent or prolonged. Insert lightly into the nostrils a small piece of cotton wool. A case in which this gave instantaneous relief, when all other remedies had failed, is recorded by Dr. Bradley. (*British Med. Jour.*, Dec. 1879.)

Spermatorrhœa. See *Seminal Discharges.*

† Carbolic Acid, as an external application in Small Pox, is strongly recommended by Dr. Aitchison. He directs that from the very earliest stage of the disease the whole body be rubbed with a mixture of the Acid (one part) and Sweet Oil (ten parts) twice daily. 'This application,' he remarks, 'relieves the patient marvellously—the oil soothing and cooling the skin, the acid deodorising the stench, and destroying the contagious influence of the particles thrown off from the skin. The oil is as much a part of the treatment as the disinfectant, and is an old Egyptian remedy for this disease. In many cases the application seems to destroy the Small Pox poison to the extent that the disease does not reach the pustular stage; the vesicles form themselves into hard lumps, dry up, and disappear, without the usual Small Pox pustular cicatrix.'

Spleen, Enlargement of, 'Ague Cake.' Give Sulphate of Iron and purgatives, as advised in Paragraph 176, or Papaw juice (296), or, better still, Cinchona Febrifuge (402). Extract of Gulancha (353) is worth a trial.†

Sprains, Blows, and Bruises. Solution of Sal Ammoniac (332), Hot Water Fomentations (393), or Evaporating Lotion (380) are most suitable applications for the early stages. Should there be much swelling and heat of skin, Leeches (212) may be necessary. When the active symptoms have subsided, Liniments of Camphor (68), Opium (291), Lemon-grass Oil (217), or Turpentine (366), are indicated. *In Sprains,* warm applications, with perfect rest of the part, are best suited for the first few days. The sprained part should be kept in a raised position, well supported, and should on no account be allowed to hang down. The following treatment is highly spoken of in cases of *Sprained Ankle.* As soon after the accident as possible immerse the foot in a tub of *hot* water for ten minutes, and then into a tub of cold water for a similar period. Afterwards put on a wet bandage pretty tight, and cover with oil-silk, plantain leaf, or other impermeable covering. *To remove subsequent swelling,* apply Alum Lotion (32). *To remove discoloration,* Solution of Sal Ammoniac (332).

† Quinine, in doses of five to eight grains thrice daily, produces the best effect in these cases; it may be advantageously combined with Sulphate of Iron (176). The most effectual local application is Biniodide of Mercury Ointment (16 grains of the Biniodide to simple Ointment, one ounce). In obstinate cases change of air is the best and only remedy.

Stiff Neck. Apply Opium Liniment (290).

Stomach, Acidity of. Give Lime Water (221). *Bleeding from.* See *Hæmorrhage from internal organs. Pains in.* See *Flatulence, Flatulent Colic, and Bowels, Spasmodic Affections of.*

Stomatitis. See *Mouth, Ulceration of.*

Sunstroke. Employ Cold Water Affusion and other measures advised in Paragraph 386. Artificial Respiration, as described in Appendix A, is worth a trial where the insensibility is deep and prolonged.

Syphilis. On the first appearance of a chancre or ulcer on the penis, sprinkle its surface with a little very finely powdered Sulphate of Iron, and this having been removed, dress subsequently with Black Wash (225) till the sore shows signs of healing. As a local application, Dr. Aitchison advocates Carbolic Acid. 'No time should be lost,' he remarks, 'in obtaining medical aid when an ulcer on the penis has formed. But when it is impossible to get such aid, touch the sore with pure Carbolic Acid, taking care that the healthy parts are not touched with it. Apply Sweet Oil to the parts after burning the ulcer, and then dress it as you would any healthy ulcer until the slough caused by the acid falls off.' Mercury (if at hand) should be given so as to induce slight soreness of the gums.† Country Sarsaparilla (163), Hydrocotyle

† To effect this, give one grain of Calomel, with a quarter or half a grain of Opium, night and morning, and should the gums at the end of a week not be affected, the dose of Calomel

(169), and Mudar (242), are better suited for the more advanced stages of the disease, or when it becomes constitutional. The use of the Country Sarsaparilla, however, may well be conjoined with the mercurial treatment from the very commencement. N.B. Avoid all the crude preparations of Mercury in use by the native doctors, or sold in the bazaars; they are likely to do incalculable mischief.

Tetanus (*Lock-jaw*). Try Datura (131). The treatment of Tetanus by smoking GUNJAH (INDIAN HEMP), introduced by Assistant-Surgeon A. C. Khastagir (*Indian Med. Gazette*, Aug. 1878), promises to supersede all others in India if it were only from the fact that the remedy is procurable at a trifling cost in every bazaar throughout the country, and that its application is simple in the extreme. A pipe, hookah, or Indian hubble-bubble, charged with about 15 grains

may be doubled. Soreness of the gums, with a peculiar (mercurial) fetor of the breath and metallic taste in the mouth, may be taken as an indication that the remedy has been carried to the required extent, and this condition it is desirable to maintain until the sore heals or the symptoms subside; this may occupy four or five weeks. No good, but rather great harm, will result from carrying the use of mercury beyond this point. Should it cause much increased flow of saliva (which is very undesirable), use the remedies advised for *Salivation*, or if during a course of mercury, the sore, instead of improving, becomes worse, it should at once be discontinued. Stimulants and all kinds of excitement, as well as exposure to atmospherical changes, especially wet, should be avoided during its use; in fact, this treatment requires the greatest care throughout, and should, if possible, be never undertaken except under proper medical supervision.

of dried Gunjah leaves, alone or mixed with twice as much tobacco leaves, is to be kept in readiness, and immediately on the indication of a spasm coming on it is to be lighted and handed to the patient with directions to smoke. By the time this is finished, or even before, the spasm relaxes, the eyes close, and the patient falls into a kind of slumber. The pipe is again charged, and kept in readiness for the approach of the next spasm, when the process is repeated with similar results. In this way the drug is administered day and night uninterruptedly, during which the irritation of the nervous system slowly but steadily yields to its influence. Mr. K. details five cases successfully treated in this manner. No auxiliary medicine, beyond an occasional purgative if required; no solid food allowed; milk and soup the only nutriments. This treatment is further advocated by Dr. J. C. Lucas, of the Bombay Medical Service (*Med. Times and Gaz.*, Feb. 21, 1880). The advantages which he claims for it are—(1) the spasms are cut short; (2) they reappear gradually at longer and longer intervals; (3) they gradually become not only less frequent, but less severe; this (4) saves the patient's vital powers, and thus, by prolonging life and preventing death, life, which would otherwise have succumbed, may eventually be saved. He places the dose at from eight to thirty grains, commencing with the smaller dose, and gradually increasing it as tolerance is established. He insists, properly, on the vast importance of quiet, perfect quiet, in a pure air (without too much breeze or draught), and he directs that the patient should on no account be disturbed to take his food or for any other reason, for which opportunity is to be taken when the patient awakes of his own accord, or from the recurrence of spasm. In the case of very young children, this mode of treatment cannot, of course, be carried out, but in all others it seems well worthy of a fair trial.

Throat, Dry and irritable states of, giving rise to cough, inhale the Vapour of Hot Decoction of Abelmoschus (3), or of Hot Water (390). *In Inflammatory states of, without Ulceration,* use the same inhalations, and allow a piece of Nitre to dissolve in the mouth (266). *Relaxed or Ulcerated Sore Throat.* Use gargles of Alum (29), Capsicum (78), Moringa (238), Black Pepper (300), or Pomegranate Rind (313). Catechu (89), Ginger (158), and Omum Seeds (316), used in substance, prove useful in some cases, as do inhalations of the vapour of Hot Vinegar (377), or simple Hot Water (390).

Tic Douloureux. See *Face Ache and Neuralgia.*

Tongue, Fissures or Cracks of, in the advanced stages of Fever, &c. Use Borax (55), or Alum (29).

Toothache sometimes yields to Opium (292*) or Catechu (89) locally applied, with or without Ginger (157), or Mustard Poultices externally. Extraction is the only certain cure in the majority of cases.

Tumours, Painful. Apply Datura in one of the forms advised in Paragraph 130, and give Opium (283) or Tincture of Datura (128) at night to procure sleep. A Tobacco leaf may often be advantageously substituted for Datura.

Ulcers may be successfully treated by the local application of solution of Sulphate of Copper (114*), Ceromel (167*), 'Oil dressing' (338), 'Water dressing'† (394), and Rice Poultices (322), varied according to circumstances; *if attended with fetid discharge*, Charcoal Poultices (91); *if with much discharge*, Catechu Ointment or Lotion (90) and Myrobalans Ointment (257). *To destroy Maggots on surface of*, Butea Seeds (65). *Sloughing, Gangrenous, or Ill-conditioned Ulcers* require Alum Ointment (31), Borax (59), Camphor (75), Ním Poultices (261), Oil of Country Nutmeg (274), Petroleum (416), Toddy Poultices (355*), Turpentine Ointment (367), Resin Ointment (372), or Sugar (410). 'Irrigation' (395) is most useful in removing the slough, and stimulating to healthy action. *If the pain and irritation are so great as to prevent sleep*, Opium (283), or Tincture of Datura (128). *To excessive Granulations* (*'Proud flesh'*), apply Sulphate of Copper (114). In all cases Country Sarsaparilla (163), Hydrocotyle (170) or Mudar (242) may advantageously be given internally; and *for Ulcers occurring in Scrofulous subjects*, Fish Liver Oil (137, 138) proves most useful.

† Dr. Aitchison states that for years he has discarded Water dressing in any form to ulcers, but has substituted for cleansing and dressing them a mixture of one part of Carbolic Acid and ten of Sweet Oil. He pronounces this a far more effectual mode of treatment.

Lime Water (224), with Fish Liver Oil (138) internally offer the best chance of success.

Vaginal Irritation is often removed, like a charm, by the application to the parts of a very weak solution of Carbolic Acid (one to 40 of Sweet Oil), if used stronger it is apt to cause great pain (*Aitchison*).

Voice, Loss of. Catechu (89), or any of the other measures directed for *Hoarseness.*

Vomiting. Amongst the remedies to allay this, are Infusion of Cloves (105), Infusion of Ginger (155), Lemon Grass Oil (216*), and Omum Water (318), with or without the addition of a little Opium (290). Apply Mustard Poultices (251), or Turpentine Stupes (362). In obstinate cases try Leeches (213). Lime Water (223*), though especially adapted for *Vomiting arising from Acidity of the Stomach,* is well worthy of a trial in all obstinate cases, especially in the *Vomiting of Infants and young children.* It is best given in milk. *Vomiting in Fevers.* Hot Water (385).

Warts seldom resist the persevering application for a week or two of Sulphate of Copper (108); a piece of it moistened should be rubbed lightly over the wart, avoiding the surrounding skin. It may be applied once every day, or every other day.

Wasps, Stings of. See *Bites, Venomous.*

Water on the Brain. See *Hydrocephalus.*

Water-brash (*Pyrosis*). Butea Gum (62), and Lime Water (223) may often be used with advantage.

Whites, See *Leucorrhœa, and Vaginal Discharges.*

Womb, Affections of. See *Uterus, Affections of.*

Worms. For Tænia, or Tape Worm, give Kamala (189), Pomegranate Root Bark (314), or Turpentine (365). When one fails another will often succeed. *For Lumbricus or Common Round Worm,* try Butea Seeds (64), Vernonia Seeds (373*b*) or Papaw Juice (295).† *For Ascarides, or Thread Worm,* use enemas of Lime Water (227), Assafœtida (36), or Turpentine (365).

Wounds, Ulcerated. See *Ulcers. Bleeding from.* See *Hæmorrhage.*

† The best remedy in these cases is SANTONIN, and considering the great prevalence of these worms amongst the people of India, and the many anomalous nervous, and other affections to which they give rise, it is advisable always to have on hand a supply of this drug. The dose for children under four years is from two to four grains; above twelve years from six to eight grains, rubbed up with about twice its weight of sugar, repeated every six or eight hours thrice in succession. A good plan is to give the Santonin at bed-time, and a small dose of Castor Oil in the morning, three days in succession. In many cases, it has been stated, no aperient is needed, one or two stools succeeding its administration containing the worms, if any are present; still it is safer to follow up its use by an aperient. It is of little or no use in Tape Worm; and in Thread Worm, though it will aid, often strikingly, in removing the worms, it will not prevent their reappearance. For Round Worm it is by far the most effectual remedy we possess.

APPENDIX A.

DIRECTIONS FOR RESTORING THE APPARENTLY DEAD FROM DROWNING.

(Reprinted by permission from the Directions issued by the Royal Humane Society.)

As soon as the body is taken out of the water, lay it on the ground, wipe it dry, and let the wind blow freely upon the surface. With this view, on no account let people crowd round the body.

The points to aimed at are—first, and immediately, the RESTORATION OF BREATHING; and secondly, after breathing is restored, the PROMOTION OF WARMTH AND CIRCULATION.

Treatment to Restore Natural Breathing.

RULE 1.—*To maintain a Free Entrance of Air into the Windpipe.*—Cleanse the mouth and nostrils;† open the mouth; draw forward the patient's tongue, and keep it forward; an elastic band over the tongue and under the chin will answer this purpose. Remove all tight clothing from about the neck and chest.

† A good plan is to turn the body gently over for a few minutes with the face to the ground, one of the hands being placed under the forehead. By this means, the water will run out of the mouth, and the tongue will fall forward, leaving the breathing opening free. On no account should the body be held up by the feet, as has been advised by some old writers.

Rule 2.—*To adjust the Patient's Position.*—Place the patient on his back on a flat surface, inclined a little from the feet upwards; raise and support the head and shoulders on a small firm cushion or folded article of dress placed under the shoulder blades.

Rule 3.—*To imitate the Movements of Breathing.*—Grasp the patient's arms just above the elbows; and draw the arms gently and steadily upwards, till they meet above the head (this is for the purpose of drawing air into the lungs), and keep the arms in that position for two seconds. Then turn down the patient's arms, and press them gently and firmly for two seconds against the sides of the chest. *See* Engravings I. and II. (This is with the object of pressing air out of the lungs. Pressure on the breast-bone will aid this.)

Repeat these measures alternately, deliberately, and perseveringly, fifteen times in a minute, until a spontaneous effort to respire is perceived, immediately upon which, cease to imitate the movements of breathing, and proceed to Induce Circulation and Warmth (*as below*).

Should a warm bath be procurable, the body may be placed in it up to the neck, continuing to imitate the movements of breathing. Raise the body in twenty seconds in a sitting position, and dash cold water against the chest and face, and pass ammonia under the nose. The patient should not be kept in the warm bath longer than five or six minutes.

Rule 4.—*To excite Inspiration.*—During the employment of the above method excite the nostrils with snuff or smelling salts, or tickle the throat with a

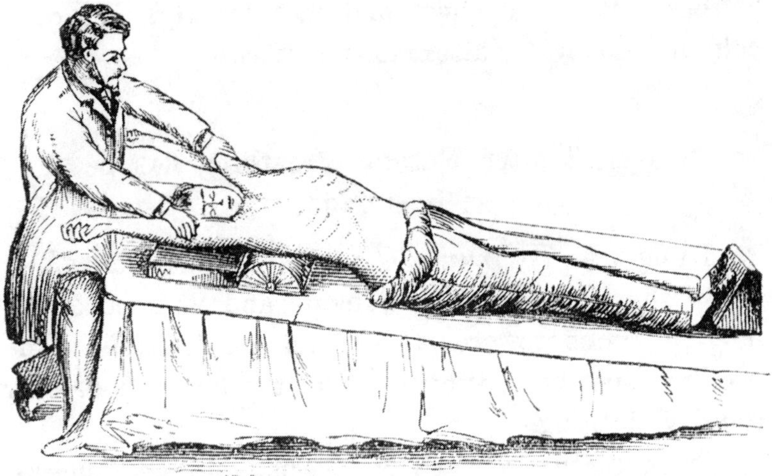

I.—Inspiration.

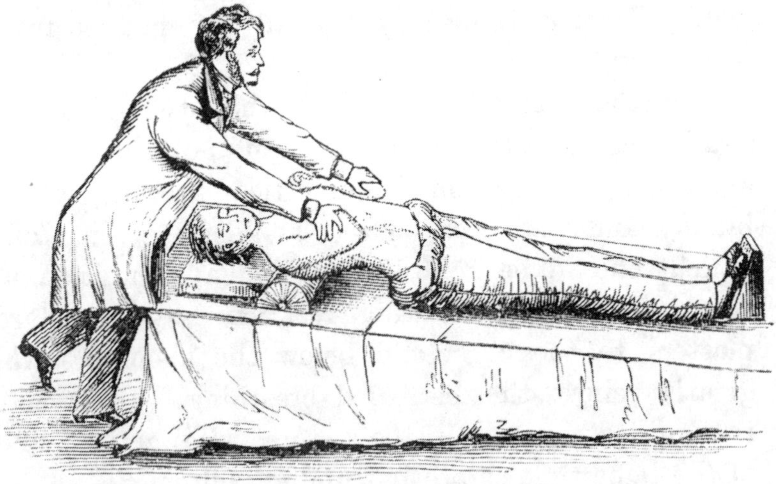

II.—Expiration.

To illustrate the position of the Body during the employment of this Method of Inducing Respiration.

feather. Rub the chest and face briskly, and dash cold and hot water alternately on them.

Treatment after Natural Breathing has been Restored.

RULE 5.—*To induce Circulation and Warmth.*—Wrap the patient in dry blankets and commence rubbing the limbs upwards, firmly and energetically. The friction must be continued under the blankets or over the dry clothing.

Promote the warmth of the body by the application of hot flannels, bottles or bladders of hot water, heated bricks, &c., to the pit of the stomach, the armpits, between the thighs, and to the soles of the feet. Warm clothing may generally be obtained from bystanders.

On the restoration of life, when the power of swallowing has returned, a teaspooonful of warm water, and subsequently small quantities of wine, warm brandy and water, or coffee, should be given. The patient should be kept in bed, and a disposition to sleep encouraged. During reaction large mustard plasters to the chest and below the shoulders will greatly relieve the distressed breathing. Great care is requisite to maintain the restored vital actions, and at the same time to prevent undue excitement.

The above treatment is to be persevered in for three or four hours, or until the pulse and breathing have ceased for at least one hour. It is an erroneous opinion that persons are irrecoverable because life does not soon make its appearance; as cases are on record of a successful result even after five hours' perseverance in the use of the above means.

APPEARANCES WHICH GENERALLY INDICATE DEATH.

There is no breathing or heart's action; the eyelids are generally half closed; the pupils dilated; the jaws clenched; the fingers semi-contracted; the tongue appearing between the teeth, and the mouth and nostrils are covered with a frothy mucus. Coldness and pallor of surface increase.

APPENDIX B.

SUMMARY OF TREATMENT OF PERSONS BITTEN BY VENOMOUS SNAKES.*

As soon as possible after a person is bitten by a snake, apply a ligature, made of a piece of cord, round the limb or part at about two or three inches above the bite.

Introduce a piece of stick or other lever between the cord and the part, and by twisting tighten the ligature to the utmost (See Stick Tourniquet, p. 215).

Apply other two or three ligatures above the first one at intervals of four or six inches, and tighten them also. After the ligature has been applied, scarify by cutting across the puncture to the depth of a quarter of an inch with a penknife or other similar cutting instrument, and let the wounds bleed freely; or better still, excise the punctured part.

Apply either a hot iron or live coal to the bottom of these wounds as quickly as possible, or some carbolic or nitric acid.

If the bite be not on a finger or toe or part where a ligature can be applied, raise up the integument with the finger and thumb, and with a sharp penknife

* Reprinted by permission from Sir Joseph Fayrer's splendid work, *The Thanatophidia of India.* Folio. London, Churchill, 1874.

cut out a circular piece as big as a finger nail round each puncture, *i.e.* round the points of the finger and thumb, to the depth of quarter to half an inch. Then apply the hot coal or hot iron to the very bottom of the wounds.

Give fifteen drops of Liquor Ammoniæ, diluted with an ounce of water, immediately, and repeat it every quarter of an hour for three or four doses, or longer, if symptoms of poisoning appear.

Or give hot brandy, or rum, or whisky, or other spirit, with an equal quantity of water, about an ounce of each (for an adult) at the same intervals.

Should no symptoms of poisoning appear in half an hour after the application of the ligatures they should be relaxed, or the part will perish from gangrene; if they should however appear, the ligatures should not be relaxed until the person be recovering from the poison, or until the ligatured part be cold and livid.

Suction of the wounds is likely to be beneficial, but as it may be dangerous to the operator, it cannot be recommended as a duty.

If, notwithstanding, symptoms of poisoning set in, and increase, if the patient become faint or depressed, unconscious, nauseated or sick, apply Mustard Poultices, or Liquor Ammoniæ on a cloth, over the stomach and heart; continue the stimulants, and keep the patient warm, but do not shut him up in a hot stifling room or small native hut—rather leave him in the fresh air than do this.

Do not make him walk about if weary or depressed,

rouse him with stimulants, mustard poultices, or ammonia, but let him rest.

If the person be first seen some time after the bite has been inflicted, and symptoms of poisoning are present, the same measures are to be resorted to. They are less likely to be successful, but nothing else can be done.

In many cases the prostration is due to fear; the bite may have been that of a harmless or exhausted snake, and persons thus bitten will rapidly recover under the use of the above measures. If poisoned, but, as is frequently the case, not fatally, these measures are the most expedient; if severely poisoned, no others are likely to be more efficacious.

People should be warned against incantations, popular antidotes, and loss of time in seeking for aid.

To the above remarks, Sir J. Fayrer adds:—'The measures suggested are no doubt severe, and not such as under other circumstances should be entrusted to non-professional persons. But the alternative is so dreadful that even at the risk of unskilful treatment, it is better that the patient should have this chance of recovery.'

Precautions to be observed by Persons residing in Snake-infested Localities.

That prevention is better than cure is admitted on all hands: hence those persons whose lot is cast in snake-infested localities will do well to lay to heart the following passage from the official 'Report on Indian and Australian Snake-poisoning,' by Drs. Joseph Ewart, Vincent Richards, and S. Coull Mackenzie (Calcutta, 1874).

The poisonous snakes of India, as a general rule, 'are, until provoked, perfectly inoffensive to all animals not required by them as food. They seldom assume the aggressive until they are rudely and accidentally disturbed. Thus a Native sleeping on the ground rolls over a venomous snake, or whilst walking in the jungle, or long grass, or in the dark, treads upon some part of a snake's body. In either case the snake bites if he can. It is in this way that a large proportion of snake accidents happen.

'A large number of lives would be saved annually if the Native population could be prevailed upon to *sleep on charpoys*, and if they got into the habit of *never stepping from their beds at night without first seeing, by means of a light, that the ground below is clear, and free from snakes.* Much of the immunity which Europeans and educated Natives enjoy from snake-bite is due to their using these very necessary precautions, especially during the rainy season, and in the mofussil by their *never walking abroad at night without a light.* There is scarcely a European of experience in the mofussil who cannot recount examples of lives (often their own) having been saved by means of these simple precautions.'

To the above judicious advice (the most important points of which I have italicised) may be added the following excellent practical precautions, communicated to me by friends whose Indian experience gives great weight to their suggestions.

1. Snakes never voluntarily traverse rough or broken ground: it is therefore advisable in snake-infested localities to surround your dwelling with a cordon or belt of broken bricks or kunkur—a breadth of three or four feet is quite sufficient for the purpose. *Dr. Norman Chevers.*

2. Be careful, especially during the wet season, to keep the verandahs, &c., free from frogs: a frog is a temptation which a snake has little or no power to resist. *Dr. Norman Chevers.* The same remark is equally applicable to rats.

3. In the cold season, if you see a snake coiled up or in an apparently lifeless state in an open well-frequented road or pathway, be careful how you approach him. Should you handle, or disturb him roughly, he will in all probability rouse up and bite you. He is only torpid from cold, not dead. *Dr. Norman Chevers.*

4. Have a piece of perforated zinc or tin fitted to the opening made for the purpose of carrying off the water out of the bath-room, if it be on the ground-floor. A similar piece should be added to the bottom of the bath-room door should it not (as

it rarely does) reach the ground beneath. *Mr. Arthur J. Waring.*

5. Discard vegetation, especially thick straggling shrubs like the Rangoon Creeper, close to your house. They are very apt to harbour snakes.

6. Important as are the above 'Precautions,' they are comparatively of small moment compared with the destruction—extermination if possible—of the snakes themselves. And this can only be efficiently carried out under Government supervision. That this is the only mode of effectually grappling with this gigantic evil, under which thousands of lives are annually sacrificed,† is forcibly set forth by Sir Joseph Fayrer, in two able papers in *Nature*, Dec. 28th, 1882, and Jan. 18th, 1883. Most earnestly is it to be hoped that Government, agreeably to his suggestion, will lose no time in establishing a department, with a responsible chief and subordinate agents, under whom a system of organized, determined, and sustained efforts for the destruction of the snakes shall be adopted and carried out. It would be a public boon if Sir Joseph's two papers were reprinted in pamphlet form and circulated throughout the length and breadth of India.

In the meanwhile zealous individual effort should be brought to bear in the same direction. To this end money rewards (heading the list with eight annas for a Cobra) should be freely offered to the Natives for every dead poisonous snake brought in, but *for*

† The numbers are 19,060 in 1880, and 18,610 in 1881, besides 4568 cattle in the two years.

poisonous ones alone. Of these there are life-like coloured plates in Fayrer's *Thanatophidia of India*; and in Ewart's *Poisonous Snakes of India*, one or other of which works is to be found in almost every large station, and which it is highly desirable for every one to make himself acquainted with. One other point remains to be noticed, namely, the necessity of carefully impounding every such dead snake brought in and paid for; otherwise it is likely to do duty a few hours later, or even next day, or it may be made the means of extracting further 'bucksheesh' from one or more of the neighbouring 'Sáhib-lóg!'

APPENDIX C.

List of articles required for carrying out the directions contained in this work :—

A set of Apothecaries' Scales and Weights (with an extra set of Weights).
1 Wedgwood Pestle and Mortar (medium size).
2 Measure Glasses (up to 6 ounces).
2 Minim Glasses.
1 Imperial Pint (20 ounces) Pewter Measure.
2 Glass Male (Urethral) Syringes.
2 Pewter ditto.
2 Glass Female (Vaginal) Syringes.
1 Metallic ditto ditto (large).
1 Enema Apparatus, fitted with metallic tubes, &c.*
1 Clinical Thermometer, with plate and some hints regarding its use.
2 Earthenware Slabs for mixing Ointments, Pills, &c.
3 Spatulas of varying length.
1 Nest of Wedgwood or Tin Funnels.
1 Nutmeg Grater.
2 Lancets in a case.
1 Sponge.
3 Yards of best Diachylon or Sticking Plaster (in tin case).

* Those with Indian-rubber or Caoutchouc flexible tubes are to be avoided, as they readily spoil in hot climates.

2 Yards of Lint.

1 Small Actual Cautery Iron. 1 Sharp Penknife or Scalpel. 6 Pieces of Whipcord.	For snake-bites, advised by Sir J. Fayrer. See Appendix B.

MEDICINES.

Sulphate of Quinine,	2 ounces.
Powdered Ipecacuanha,	8 ,,
Calomel,	4 ,,
Biniodide of Mercury,	4 ,,
Santonin,	4 ,,
Bromide of Potassium,	4 ,,
Acetate of Lead,	8 ,,

Opium (in 1 grain pills), No. 200
,, in Laudanum, 8 ounces.

Blistering Fluid. (Liquor Epispasticus, *Brit. Ph.*)	4 ounces.

Liquor Ammoniæ, 8 ounces.
Carbolic Acid, 2 pints.

N.B.—These should be kept in well glass-stoppered or well-corked bottles, and protected, as far as possible, from the action of light and heat.

INDEX OF ARTICLES.